GW01311313

With Outstretched Arms

A 40-Day Inspirational Devotional for Health Care Workers and Caregivers

Josephine V. Corriette, RN

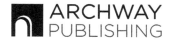

Copyright © 2019 Josephine V. Corriette, RN.

All rights reserved. No part of this book may be used or reproduced by any means, graphic, electronic, or mechanical, including photocopying, recording, taping or by any information storage retrieval system without the written permission of the author except in the case of brief quotations embodied in critical articles and reviews.

Archway Publishing books may be ordered through booksellers or by contacting:

Archway Publishing
1663 Liberty Drive
Bloomington, IN 47403
www.archwaypublishing.com
1 (888) 242-5904

Because of the dynamic nature of the Internet, any web addresses or links contained in this book may have changed since publication and may no longer be valid. The views expressed in this work are solely those of the author and do not necessarily reflect the views of the publisher, and the publisher hereby disclaims any responsibility for them.

Any people depicted in stock imagery provided by Getty Images are models, and such images are being used for illustrative purposes only.
Certain stock imagery © Getty Images.

Scripture quotations marked (NIV) are taken from the Holy Bible, New International Version®, NIV®. Copyright © 1973, 1978, 1984, 2011 by Biblica, Inc.™ Used by permission of Zondervan. All rights reserved worldwide. www.zondervan.com The "NIV" and "New International Version" are trademarks registered in the United States Patent and Trademark Office by Biblica, Inc.™

Scripture taken from the New King James Version®. Copyright © 1982 by Thomas Nelson. Used by permission. All rights reserved.

Scripture taken from the King James Version of the Bible.

ISBN: 978-1-4808-8494-6 (sc)
ISBN: 978-1-4808-8495-3 (e)

Library of Congress Control Number: 2019918036

Print information available on the last page.

Archway Publishing rev. date: 11/21/2019

Presented to:

_____

From:

_____

ACKNOWLEDGMENTS

Thank You Dear Lord for providing an opportunity to minister to others throughout my lifetime. I dedicate this book to You.

To my late mother, Edith G. Mills, a stalwart for Jesus, prayed unceasingly for me. I pray that her legacy lives on through me.

To my husband, Vansley, thank you for keeping me grounded and for your culinary skills that have allowed me more time to write this devotional. Also, special thanks to my daughter, Allison, for her continued help and support to make this devotional, *With Outstretched Arms*, a reality. Sincerest thanks to my son, Ben, for his insight and prayers. To Donovan, my grandson, thank you for giving me ideas and suggestions; you are special indeed.

Introduction

To God be the glory for all He has done and continues to do. I've had the privilege of writing personal journals for many years during reading, meditation, and prayer. God has given me many sermons and words of encouragement and hope, which I have written down and shared with you in this book.

In this inspirational devotional, *With Outstretched Arms,* I've prayerfully included 40 prayers, health nuggets, hope and prosperity gems, and a few of my poems to encourage you in the Lord. After much prayer, the Lord reminded me of the significance of the number 40. It is repeated several times in the Bible; 40 represents judgment and ministry: Moses led the children of Israel out of Egyptian bondage but they journeyed 40 years in the wilderness because of their rebellion; Jesus spent 40 days with His disciplines after His resurrection and fasted for 40 days in the wilderness before He began His public ministry.

May God continue to bless you and your clients. You are indeed special to God; He loves you with an everlasting and steadfast love. Blessings to you now and always. You are loved.

Day 1

Come unto Me and Rest

> Come unto me, all ye that labour and are heavy laden, and I will give you rest. Take my yoke upon you, and learn of me; for I am meek and lowly in heart: and ye shall find rest unto your souls. For my yoke is easy, and my burden is light.
>
> —Matthew 11:28–30 (KJV)

Mary, a hard-working health care professional, never appeared tired or listless, even after working very long hours. She seldom took required breaks and never disclosed the problems and concerns that overwhelmed her. Day after day, week after week, year after year, Mary continued this vigorous, life-draining routine. Unfortunately, she started exhibiting fatigue and unsteady gait, resulting in her inability to work. Numerous diagnostic tests failed to detect any physiological cause. She was eventually diagnosed with severe stress and anxiety, which resulted in the shut-down of her neurological function. She was eventually confined to a wheelchair.

The same is true when we try to carry all of our cares and burdens without the aid of the Holy Spirit and the source of life and strength, the Lord Jesus. In order for you to function optimally, you must cast your burdens on the Lord, for He promises to sustain and help you. Moreover, the Lord says:

> Be careful for nothing; but in everything by prayer and supplication with thanksgiving let your requests be made known unto God. And the peace of God, which passeth all understanding, shall keep your hearts and minds through Christ Jesus. (Philippians 4:6–7 KJV)

So as you rest in the Lord, you'll be able to find the comfort and rest you need.

A Prayer for Today
Dear Heavenly Father, I feel very stressed and anxious at times. Please help me to lay all my burdens at the foot of the cross and leave them there. Please fill me with Your peace and joy, in the name of Jesus. Amen.

Health Nugget
Take time out of your busy schedule to relax and smell the roses. You are worth it.

Hope and Prosperity Gem
You need not worry or fret. Just relax in the everlasting arms of God, and He will give you peace and rest to your soul.

Cast Your Cares upon the Master

Cast your cares upon the Master,
for you'll find peace and rest.
Cast your love a little faster,
and you'll receive God's best.

Cast your burdens at the foot of the cross,
for you'll find guidance.
Cast yourself at the feet of Jesus, and in Him be lost,
and you'll find deliverance.

Day 2

Jesus Is Full of Compassion

> So He answered and said, "You shall love the Lord your God with all your heart, with all your soul, with all your strength, and with all your mind, and your neighbor as yourself."
>
> —Luke 10:27 (NKJV)

Mrs. Zella, a health care professional, believed in delivering excellent care to all her clients, regardless of their demeanor. One of her clients, however, was rude and offensive toward her. Mrs. Zella said an earnest prayer, and God gave her the wisdom and understanding she needed to minister and care for the client effectively.

The next day, to her surprise, the client invited her into his room and earnestly apologized for his uncouth behavior. He even asked her to pray for him because he felt so much better when she did. This client eventually gave his heart to the Lord; he also attended church and was active in ministry.

Mrs. Zella's experience solidified her commitment to always provide loving care to all her clients, regardless of their attitudes. Mrs. Zella treated everyone with love and respect. This caring attitude had an indelible influence on her coworkers and the interdisciplinary team.

Likewise, the story of the Good Samaritan in Luke 10:33–37 (KJV) shows us a man who was compassionate to a total stranger who was injured by thieves and left half-dead on the road. Verses 33–37 declare:

> But a certain Samaritan, as he journeyed, came where he was: and when he saw him, he had compassion on him, and went to him, and bound up his wounds, pouring in oil and wine, and set him on his own beast, and brought him to an inn, and took care of him. And on the morrow when he departed, he took out two pence, and gave them to the host, and said unto him, take care of him; and whatsoever thou spendest more, when I come again, I will repay thee.

The moral of the story is that you should lay aside differences and help those who are in need. The Samaritan was not concerned about the injured person's religion or race; he saw an injured man, showed mercy, and provided compassionate care. Likewise, the Lord is calling us to show empathy and kindness.

A Prayer for Today
Dear Lord, please help us to show compassion to those in need and do so with a heart of love and mercy. We are indeed our brother's keeper, so help us to love our neighbor as ourselves in the name of Jesus. Amen.

Health Nugget
Share health and wellness principles as the need arises. Live each day to the fullest, and never let go of your integrity.

Hope and Prosperity Gem

God is a God of compassion who takes care of all He has made. As we do the same, we'll enjoy the peace of the Lord and abundant life. He will also bless you when you take the time to show compassion to those in need. So let's do likewise.

Storehouse of God's Grace and Mercy

We are storehouses of God's grace and mercy;
His compassion fails not.
It's new every morning, He taught,
and for our welfare and safety, He sought.

We're not consumed because of His mercy;
His love is immeasurable.
His grace is unsearchable,
and His compassion indescribable.

Day 3

Rich Blessing of the Lord

The blessing of the Lord makes one rich, and He adds no sorrow with it.

—Proverbs 10:22 (NKJV)

Do you know that God wants you to prosper, and be healthy, and enjoy a victorious life? Are you anticipating an abundant life filled with His rich blessings? Additionally, the Lord's blessings are His original plan for you. As you do good, show mercy, and help the poor and needy, the favor of the Lord will be evident in your life. Love as the Lord loves, and learn to forgive as He forgives.

> And whatsoever ye do, do it heartily, as to the Lord, and not unto men; Knowing that of the Lord ye shall receive the reward of the inheritance: for ye serve the Lord Christ. (Colossians 3:23–24 KJV)

> Therefore, all things whatsoever ye would that men should do to you, do ye even so to them: for this is the law and the prophets. (Matthew 7:12 KJV)

Whether you are dealing with a difficult client or a loved one, provide excellent care. Do it with a heart full of love. After you have done the best you can, you'll experience a sense of satisfaction and contentment.

God's Word affirms in Psalm 84:11–12 KJV, "For the LORD God is a sun and shield: the LORD will give grace and glory: no good thing will he withhold from them that walk uprightly. O LORD of hosts, blessed is the man that trusteth in thee."

A Prayer for Today
Dear Lord, thank You for the opportunity to take good care of my clients in Your Name. Help me always to work as unto You. Then my reward will be sure.

Health Nugget
When you give with a willing heart, you'll enjoy health and peace.

Hope and Prosperity Gem
Whatever you do, do it with a willing heart. Treat others well, and God's abundant blessings will follow you. "For You, O Lord, will bless the righteous; with favor, You will surround him as with a shield" (Psalm 5:12 KJV).

Do Not Be Covetous

Do not be covetous.
Be content and not envious,
for that's your eye salve
and will prolong your days.

A man's life consists not in the abundance
of the things he possesses but needs temperance;
as you trust in God with a thankful heart,
He'll give you good things to enjoy that'll never depart.

Thank You, Heavenly Father,
for Your many blessings to gather.
Your handiwork is all over me,
and Your rich blessings for all to see.

We Come into Your Presence

We come into Your presence with hands lifted high.
We come into Your presence with voices lifted high.
We come into Your presence with songs of praise.
We come into Your presence with hearts full of praise.

Lord, Your blessings will come down,
as we praise You; yes, the blessings will come down.
We glorify, adore, and worship You.
We love, magnify, and reverence You.

Day 4

A Land Flowing with Milk and Honey

And my God will supply all your needs according to His riches in glory by Christ Jesus.

—Philippians 4:19 (NKJV)

Moses, the man of God, rehearsed in the hearing of all the children of Israel the things God had done for them as they were about to possess the Promised Land, Canaan. It was a fertile land with much wealth and precious stones, and flowing with milk and honey. The Lord gave them bread from heaven, and the Ten Commandments written with His own finger. Additionally, He protected them from their enemies.

Unfortunately, they provoked the Lord to anger because of their disobedience and idolatry. The Lord wanted to destroy them, but Moses fell on his knees and interceded for them. God answered his prayers and did not destroy them. We serve a merciful and long-suffering God Who does not treat us as we deserve.

Similarly, the Lord wants us to learn from their experiences: "Trust in the Lord with all thine heart; and lean not unto thine own understanding. In all thy ways acknowledge him, and he shall direct thy paths" (Proverbs 3:5–6 KJV).

God's mercy endures to all generations. He loves you with an everlasting and steadfast love and holds you with His righteous right hand. Hold on to Jesus, for He is holding on to you. Moreover, Philippians 4:19 (KJV) states, "But my Lord will supply all your needs according to His riches in glory by Christ Jesus the Lord. You don't need to worry." 1 Corinthians 2:9 (NIV) declares, "Eye has not seen, nor ear heard, nor have entered into the heart of man, the things which God has prepared for those who love Him. Therefore, no matter what you are going through, God is there with you and will take care of you." All your needs He will supply because He is Jehovah Jireh. Trust and obey Him.

A Prayer for Today: Thank You, Lord, for Your mercy and grace. You have not treated me as I deserve but have lavished me with Your love and compassion. Thank You for supplying all my needs according to Your riches in glory by Christ Jesus, the Lord. Amen.

Health Nugget: Give thanks to the Lord with a grateful and merry heart, for it is an effective medicine.

Hope and Prosperity Gem: Do good to all, especially to the poor and needy, and the Lord will reward you with abundant blessings. Additional blessings could be yours, if you fear and reverence Him.

Sow Bountifully, Reap Abundantly

Sow bountifully, reap abundantly,
sow sparingly, reap meagerly.
Give cheerfully, receive plentifully,
give grudgingly, receive scantily.

Give of necessity or compulsion, no blessing you'll receive
but curse and expulsion, so don't be deceived.
Give willingly, and God will supply all your needs;
therefore, be obedient to Him and plant your seeds.

All Your Needs He'll Supply

All your needs He'll supply, for on Him you can rely.
Don't be discouraged, for Jesus hears your cry.
He sees every teardrop and hears your earnest prayers.
So hope in God, for He'll wipe away all your tears.

Day 5

You're Never Alone, for God Is with You

> Have I not commanded you? Be strong and courageous. Do not be afraid; do not be discouraged, for the Lord your God will be with you wherever you go.
>
> —Joshua 1:9 (NIV)

You are never alone, for God is with you in the good times and the bad. When you feel that you can't continue for another second because of the difficulties and challenges of being a health care worker or caregiver, don't give up.

The burdens of life are not uncommon. Job 14:1–2 (KJV) declares, "Man that is born of a woman is of few days and full of trouble. He cometh forth like a flower, and is cut down: he fleeth also as a shadow, and continueth not." That's why we must love one another, even as the Lord loves us. Everyone is valuable in the sight of God. Thus, let's treat each other with honor and respect, realizing that we are all brothers and sisters in Christ.

God's promises are true. He promises that He will never leave you nor forsake you. You may feel all alone, and you may be experiencing the loss of a loved one, unemployment, difficulty on the job, unfair or unequal treatment, loneliness, divorce, or some other source of unhappiness. Remember that God loves you unconditionally, and nothing in this world or the next will ever separate you from His love.

Apostle Paul, in Romans 8:35…38–39 (KJV), states, "Who shall separate us from the love of Christ? Shall tribulation, or distress, or persecution, or famine, or nakedness, or peril, or sword? For I am persuaded, that neither death, nor life, nor angels, nor principalities, nor powers, nor things present, nor things to come, nor height, nor depth, nor any other creature, shall be able to separate us from the love of God, which is in Christ Jesus our Lord."

As you rest in the sheltering arms of the Lord, you will find peace and rest. God is good, and His mercy endures forever.

When you've worked untiringly and have gone beyond the call of duty but still receive a pink slip, indicating that your services are no longer needed, that is disheartening. The pain of rejection is real, but the blood of Jesus can heal your wounded soul. Therefore, you must run to Jesus and cry out to Him to give you the strength and courage to cope. The Lord will comfort you and speak sweet words of acceptance and love.

In times of difficulty, you need a Savior Who always embraces you. That One is Jesus, the lover of your soul. He will never leave you nor forsake you, so you may boldly say, "The Lord is my Helper, and I will not fear what man shall do unto me" (Hebrews 13:6 KJV). You have nothing to fear, for God is sheltering you under His wings.

God is preparing you for something bigger and better. He is just making room for you to expand your employment, ministry, and influence. As the apostle Paul declares in Ephesians 6:10–11 (KJV), "Finally, my brethren, be strong in the Lord, and in the power of his might. Put on the whole armour of God, that ye may be able to stand against the wiles of the devil." Hold on to Jesus, for He is holding on to you. He will make a way and reward you with favor and blessings.

Prayer for Today: Dear Lord, thank You for being my very present help in times of trouble. Thank You for loving me with an everlasting love. I am not alone, for You are with me wherever I go. Amen.

Health Nugget: Rest securely in the loving arms of Jesus and let His peace and joy flow through you.

Hope and Prosperity Gem: If God is for you, who can ever be against you? God is fighting your battles; stand still, and see the deliverance of the Lord.

You Are Not Alone

You are not alone,
when temptation overtakes you;
for this is common to man.
Just like grains of sand.

You are not alone,
when temptation crosses your path.
God is faithful, and He'll help you
and make a way of escape too.
You are not alone.

When temptation raises its ugly head,
look to Jesus, for He said,
I will never leave you nor forsake you,
for His blood He shed.

You are not alone,
when temptation comes.
God is faithful and will not give you more than you can bear.
For He's there to help you.
You are not alone.

Day 6

Paralyzed by Fear

> Be anxious for nothing, but in everything by prayer and supplication, with thanksgiving, let your requests be made known to God; and the peace of God which surpasses all understanding, will guard your hearts and minds through Christ Jesus.
>
> —Philippians 4:6 (NKJV)

You don't need to be paralyzed by fear of the unknown. God has already gone before you to clear the way. There is no need to worry, and there is no need to fret because He has never failed you yet. So many blessings and abundant living have slipped from the hands of God's children because of fear and unbelief. May God help us today. Dear Lord, please alleviate our disbelief.

Moses died on Mount Nebo, just as the Lord foretold. He did not enter the land flowing with milk and honey because he struck the rock in anger instead of speaking to it, as God had commanded. Moses called the Hebrews rebels because of their constant murmuring and complaining. The rock represented Jesus, the Rock of Ages, the Bright and Morning Star.

As health care workers and caregivers, let us always look to the author and finisher of our faith, Jesus. Fear and anxiety will not touch you if you lean on the arms of Jesus and cast all your cares upon Him. His arms are not too short that He cannot heal; He is willing and able to remove all your doubts and fears. Never again will you be paralyzed by fear, if you believe by faith. 2 Timothy 1:17 (KJV) says, "God has not given you a spirit of fear but a spirit of love, of power, and a sound mind."

Look fear in the eye and say: "Fear, I come against you in the name of Jesus; you have no authority over me, for God has given me the power to overcome you, and I will walk in boldness and victory.

A Prayer for Today: Dear Lord, You have not given me a spirit of fear but a sound mind and a spirit of power and of love. Help me always to remember that You are comforting and holding me in Your loving arms; therefore, I have nothing to fear. Amen.

Health Nugget: Take a ten-minute nap in the afternoon; this may help with good health and longevity.

Hope and Prosperity Gem: Do not be paralyzed by fear because God has not given you a spirit of fear or timidity but of power and self-discipline.

Fear and Anxiety

Fear and anxiety can paralyze.
Fear and anxiety immobilize.

Don't let fear keep you down.
Rise up and let your mind be sound.
Shake off the dust from under your feet
and sound aloud Satan's defeat.

The charge I give is from God's Word.
Use your Bible as your sword.
For in it, fear and anxiety do not exist.
So put on God's armor, and you'll be fit.

Face Fear Head On

Face fear head on.
Face it like a man.
Face it like a woman,
and face it like God's Son.

Tackle fear on your knees.
Pray to God for help, for He sees.
Believe His Word and in faith firmly stand
and receive your deliverance.

Day 7

Don't Lose Hope

> If my people, which are called by my name, shall humble themselves, and pray, and seek my face, and turn from their wicked ways; then will I hear from heaven, and will forgive their sin, and will heal their land.
>
> —2 Chronicles 7:14 (KJV)

Hold on to Jesus, for He is holding on to you. No good things will He hold back from them who walk in sincerity and truth. So, "what shall we then say to these things? If God be for us, who can be against us?" Romans 8:31 (KJV).

> "Ye are of God, little children, and have overcome them: because greater is He that is in you, than He that is in the world" (1 John 4:4 KJV).

> "But if you bite and devour one another, beware lest you be consumed by one another" (Galatians 5:15 NKJV).

The prophet Moses is an example of someone who showed love instead of hate and humility instead of arrogance. He did not fight or quarrel for the highest position. Even though he was taunted and disrespected at times by the Hebrews, he kept his focus and trust in the Lord of Abraham, Isaac, and Jacob. He never gave up but remained faithful and unmovable in the work of God.

So don't give up. When things get tough and challenging to manage, remember Moses. God is a good God. He still has work for you to do, so keep on going until you can go no more. Once you have life, you can work for the Lord in big or small ways. What a mighty God we serve. Our service for the Lord is never in vain.

"When thou hast eaten and art full, then thou shalt bless the Lord thy God for the good land which he hath given thee. But thou shalt remember the Lord thy God: for it is he that giveth thee power to get wealth, that he may establish his covenant which he sware unto thy fathers, as it is this day" (Deuteronomy 8:10, 18 KJV). "And whatsoever ye do in word or deed, do all in the name of the Lord Jesus, giving thanks to God and the Father by him" (Colossians 3:17 KJV).

Enjoy the victorious life God has ordained for you. Trust and obey, and He'll make a way for you. Moreover, never give up but keep holding onto Jesus, for He is holding on to you.

I've known many health care professionals who have given up their wholesome careers because of unfair treatment by administrators and coworkers alike. Several of them have chosen other jobs. However, diligence, persistence, commitment, and hard work are key ingredients needed for success and happiness.

Many have chosen the easy and broad way, which will ultimately lead to destruction, but few have chosen the narrow way. "Because strait is the gate, and narrow is the way, which leadeth unto life, and few there be that find it" (Matthew 7:14 KJV). So stay on the narrow road, and do not veer off; this may be the road God has ordained for you to travel. Matthew 24:13 (KJV) also declares, "But he that shall endure unto the end, the same shall be saved."

Those who continue to work for the Lord will also receive a crown of life. So hang in there and trust God, and He will help you to stay the course.

A Prayer for Today: Father, I bow in Your Holy presence, fill me with the power of the Holy Spirit. Help me never to give up but keep my eyes on You. Amen.

Health Nugget: Breathe fresh air into your lungs, and enjoy God's beautiful creation.

Hope and Prosperity Gem: True love makes the world go around and can allow you to live a happy and prosperous life as you surrender all to Jesus.

Don't Lose Hope, Don't Give Up

When you feel so all alone,
with no friends to call your own,
remember Jesus cares and understands.
He'll guide and keep you through the deserted lands.

When you feel that all hope is gone,
remember God is always by your side.
Jesus cares and understands,
and with you He'll abide.

When you feel like giving up,
remember God has the cup,
the cup of healing and deliverance,
for He knows your circumstance.

Don't lose hope, but cry out to Jesus.
He'll help you cope, and your eyes won't be dim.
Yes, Jesus will rescue you, for He's Jesus, our King.
So let's shout praises and sing to Him.

What Would Jesus Do?

What would Jesus do, if you were hurting?
What would Jesus do, if you were lonely?
What would Jesus do, if no one loved you?
What would Jesus do, if you were hungry?

Jesus would embrace you, if you were hurting.
Jesus would speak words of hope and comfort, if you were lonely.
Jesus would show you His steadfast, everlasting love.
Jesus would provide you with more than enough grace from above.

Jesus is a Friend who sticks closer than a brother,
a Friend of sinners of whom I am chief.
Jesus died so that you'd not have to suffer,
a Friend of sinners who died between two thieves.

That's what Jesus would do:
He'd heal the sick and raise the dead,
and walk on water to aid you,
plus preach the Gospel as He said.

Day 8

Your Labor Is Not in Vain

> For God is not unjust to forget your work and labor of love which you have shown toward His name, in that you have ministered to the saints, and do minister.
>
> —Hebrew 6:10 (NKJV)

Do not labor to be wealthy, for riches have wings, and they usually fly away. Likewise, "Do not labor for the food which perishes, but for the food which endures to everlasting life, which the Son of God will give you, because God the Father has set His seal on Him" (John 6:27 NKJV). "For all the promises of God in him are yea, and in him Amen, unto the glory of God by us" (2 Corinthians 1:20 KJV).

"Therefore if thine enemy hunger, feed him; if he thirst, give him drink: for in so doing thou shalt heap coals of fire on his head. Be not overcome of evil, but overcome evil with good" (Romans 12:20 KJV).

As you face the rigor of the day, angels are shielding you, as is the God of the universe. You may be harassed today by the enemy, but remember who is on your side; God is on your side. The Bible says, "He that dwelleth in the secret place of the Most High shall abide under the shadow of the Almighty. I will say of the Lord, He is my refuge and my fortress: my God in Him I will trust" (Psalm 91:1-2 KJV).

David also affirms this in Psalm 46:1 (NKJV): "The Lord is our refuge and strength, a very present help in trouble." You have nothing to fear. God admonishes you to stand still, and you'll see how He'll work everything out for your good. You may not understand why you are experiencing hardship. Notwithstanding, God said that no good thing would He withhold from you if you love Him and walk uprightly.

Nothing that you are going through now is beyond the scope of God's power and sovereignty. Stand still, and watch what the Lord will do. Be content with what you have, for this is God's will for you in Christ Jesus. Jesus declares in 2 Corinthians 12:9 (KJV), "My grace is sufficient for thee: for my strength is made perfect in weakness."

"Nay in all these things we are more than conquerors through Him that loves us" (Romans 8:37 KJV). More than this, the battle is not yours; it's the Lord's. Hold on to Jesus, for He's holding on to you. You can be confident of His promises. Go and do what the Lord wants you to do. The Lord has your back and is working on your behalf, even though the staff is not.

A Prayer for Today: Dear Father, fill my life with good works so that people will glorify and magnify Your Holy name, in Jesus' Holy name, I pray. Amen.

Health Nugget: Try to get at least eight hours of sleep daily; this will help to restore your energy levels and repair the vital organs in your body.

Hope and Prosperity Gem: Always give yourself entirely to the work of the Lord, because you know that your labor is not in vain. "Delight thyself also in the Lord and He shall give thee the desires of thine heart" (Psalm 37:4 KJV).

God Will Not Forget Your Labor of Love

God is not unrighteous to forget your labor of love.
Your service for Him will be recorded above.

Come and do the work God has called you to do.
Come and love, for He has His hand on you.

Don't be afraid of the unknown,
for He's our High Priest seated on the throne.

Day 9

Do Good Like Jesus

Therefore be imitators of God, as beloved children.

—Ephesians 5:1 (NKJV)

God admonishes us to do good and live a life of obedience, like Jesus. When Jesus was on earth, He loved the unlovable, raised the dead, preached, taught about the kingdom of heaven, and lived a holy and perfect life. He set for us an example to continue to work for Him.

Just like Jesus did good throughout His ministry on earth, He will equip us to do the same. Romans 12 (KJV) tells us to "let love be without dissimulation. Abhor that which is evil; cleave to that which is good. Recompense to no man evil for evil. Provide things honest in the sight of all men. If it be possible, as much as lieth in you, live peaceably with all men. Be not overcome of evil, but overcome evil with good."

The task to do good in this sinful world is difficult without the aid of the Holy Spirit. That's why we must commit our lives to Jesus and ask Him to help us to do good, as He did.

As you dedicate your life to the Lord and walk in His footsteps, you'll enjoy a fruitful life. Galatians 5:22-23 (KJV) declares, "But the fruit of the Spirit is love, joy, peace, longsuffering, gentleness, goodness, faith, Meekness, temperance: against such there is no law."

When you walk in the Spirit, all these virtues will be evident in your life as you purpose in your heart to do good. James 4:17 (KJV) says, "Therefore to him that knoweth to do good and doeth it not, to him it is sin."

Whether you labor in the medical field, at home, in the church, or even in the mission field as a health care worker, remember whatever you do, do it as unto the Lord.

A Prayer for Today: Dear God, please help me to do good like Jesus and to be an example to those around me so I can bring honor and glory to Your Holy name. Help me also to live in faith and obedience to the name of Jesus. Amen.

Health Nugget: Be kind to yourself and others. Help those who are less fortunate. Furthermore, make better food choices; reduce sugar, salt, and fat in your diet. Also, take time to enjoy nature, and take deep cleansing breaths throughout the day.

Hope and Prosperity Gem: When you give generously and do good to the less fortunate, you're honoring God, their Maker. It is a sin to despise one's neighbor, but blessed is the one who is kind to the poor and needy. Proverbs 11:25 (KJV) says that "the liberal soul shall be made fat: and he that watereth shall be watered also himself."

Lifestyle of Obedience

Living a lifestyle of obedience
is just common sense,
but learn to lean on Jesus,
for He's the example that God sent.

A strong desire of Christ to follow
will avoid a life that's hollow.
A lifestyle of obedience to beset
is just common decency and respect.

God is an Awesome God
to cherish and to love,
to worship and to call Him Lord,
that's what He's worthy of.

Learn submission.
Be willing to do what He wants you to do.
Practice proactive contrition.
Be willing to do what God wants you to do.

Following Jesus is a wise decision,
and acknowledging Him as Lord of your life
will help you avoid derision.
So say yes to Jesus Christ.

Day 10

Hold on to Jesus

> Let us hold fast the profession of our faith without wavering; for he is faithful that promised.
>
> —Hebrews 10:23 (KJV)

You'll reap a harvest if you don't give up. Be encouraged today, for your labor is not in vain in the Lord. You may feel downtrodden and defeated, but do not be dismayed or discouraged, for the Lord promises to help you and strengthen you.

Look not at your situation, but look to Jesus. Focus on Him, and He will hold you with His mighty right hand. Little is plenty, if the Lord is in it. Do not labor for wealth or uncertain riches. Work to the honor and glory of the Lord.

Use your gifts and talents to bring glory and praise to the Lord, and never be afraid. God has given you the power to do great and wonderful things for Him. Surrender your life and dreams to Him today. The Bible clearly states that He has given you a spirit of power and love and a sound mind to worship Him and love your brothers and sisters.

You are also admonished to love your neighbor as yourself and treat them with love and respect. Show mercy and be humble. God cannot walk with the proud or the scornful.

I remember an incident with a caregiver who was very arrogant and thought she knew everything. She would ridicule everyone and refused to take advice, even from the physicians. It didn't take long before she had to humble herself because she lost almost everything.

The Lord says that the haughty spirit will cause you to fall. So be humble and kind. The Lord promises us in Matthew 7:7 (KJV), "Ask, and it shall be given you; seek, and ye shall find; knock, and it shall be opened unto you." If we ask in faith according to His will, God will answer our prayers.

Therefore, do not be afraid of the dark, for Jesus is with you everywhere you go. His protecting angels are there to help us. A few years ago, I needed help to lift a patient back into the wheelchair. It was drizzling outside, so I said a prayer in my heart. Before I could call for help, a young man holding an umbrella walked toward us, lifted the patient, and placed him in the wheelchair, without difficulty. He then pushed him up the ramp to the main door and then disappeared. Yes, I still believed he was my guardian angel. I will never forget that incident. God is a good God, for He's always taking care of His children.

Health care personnel and caregivers, do not be afraid, for God loves you with endless love. Lean on His comforting, outstretched arms.

A Prayer for Today: When I am afraid, I will trust in You, O Lord. Please continue to hold my right hand with Your righteous right hand. I love You, Lord; help me to put my trust and confidence in You and live a victorious life.

Health Nugget: Wait on the Lord, and be of good courage, and He will strengthen your heart; wait, I say, on the Lord of glory. Enjoy the journey. Be not afraid but be of good cheer.

Hope and Prosperity Gem: Don't be afraid, but do what the Lord has asked you to do. He will give you the ability and strength to do the work He calls you to do. When the Lord calls you, He empowers you and equips you.

Don't Be Afraid, for God Is with You

Don't be afraid, for as long as the earth remains,
seedtime and harvest, cold and heat,
winter and summer, day and night will not cease.
The Lord is pleading for us at the Mercy Seat.

So don't be afraid, for God is with you.
For the Word of God will abide forever,
heaven and earth will pass away,
but God's love will not sever.

Thank You, Lord

My pen and ink cannot express my gratitude
to my Maker and my King,
for He's the One Who gives me latitude
to praise Him, worship Him, and to Him I sing.

Lord, You are incredible.
You are touched with the feelings
of my infirmities.
Lord, You are incredible.

Don't Be Afraid to Use Your Gifts and Talents

God placed us on earth with gifts and talents
to be used since birth, in order for our lives to be balanced.
Our gifts and talents should benefit everyone around us,
so that the world will be a better place as we adjust.

Don't wait to be appointed.
Don't be afraid, just volunteer your services,
and you won't be disappointed.
But be aware of Satan's cunning tricks and devices.

Remember in Christ, you can do all things.
His strength and peace He will give.
Do your work with dignity and without strings.
Don't be afraid; believe in His power to love and forgive.

Day 11

Stand Still

> And Moses said unto the people, fear not, stand still, and see the salvation of the Lord, which He will shew to you today: for the Egyptians whom ye have seen, ye shall see no more forever.
>
> —Exodus 14:13 (KJV)

Exodus 14 tells of the crossing of the Red Sea. The children of Israel were terrified of the Egyptian army that pursued them. God commanded Moses to stretch forth his rod over the Red Sea so that the children of Israel could cross over on dry land.

The following day, the bodies of the Egyptian army washed up on the seashore; they all drowned. God is faithful, so be not afraid. He will take care of you and make your enemies your footstool.

A health care worker was afraid to lose her job. She was always jittery and fearful. However, she was a diligent and conscientious worker. At times, she would cry and say, "I'm a single mom and cannot afford to lose my job." She would repeat the following statements several times a week: "If I lose my job, how could I take care of my children? I'm a single mother trying to make ends meet." She seemed afraid of everything. Any reports of instability in the job market would make her cry.

Everyone assured this health care worker that she was doing an excellent job. After much encouragement and assurance from the staff, along with fervent prayers, she eventually accepted the fact that her job was secure and not in jeopardy. She continued providing excellent care to all her clients and expressed gratitude for everyone's kindness and love. James 5:16 (KJV) asserts that "the effectual prayer of a righteous man availeth much."

Here are the encouraging words of the apostle Paul in Philippians 4:6–7 (KJV): "Be anxious for nothing, but in everything by prayer and supplication, with thanksgiving, let your requests be made known to God, and the peace of God, which surpasses all understanding, will guard your hearts and minds through Christ Jesus."

A Prayer for Today: Help me, Lord, to stand firm and still, and see Your salvation and deliverance. Thank You for Your faithfulness and love. Amen.

Health Nugget: In everything, give thanks to the Lord, for this is His will concerning you. Laugh a lot and be happy. It's terrific for your health and well-being.

Hope and Prosperity Gem: Stand still, and see the salvation of the Lord. Win your battle on your knees in prayer, and see God turn your anxieties and problems into joy.

Don't Retire from Living

Don't retire from living
but retire from a life of sin;
Continue thriving and living,
and as you witness, be a soul-winner for Him.

Stand fast.
Stand firm.
Don't be afraid,
for Jesus will be your aid.

I Dare to Be Different

I dare to be different,
in a world of compromise.
I dare to be different,
even though they tell many lies.

I dare to be different,
when people do as they please.
I dare to be different,
even though they may tease.

I dare to be different
and stand up for the right.
I dare to be different,
even though they're out of sight.

Day 12

God Restores

> And I will restore to you the years that the locust hath eaten, the cankerworm, and the caterpillar, and the palmerworm, my great army which I sent among you. You will eat in plenty and be satisfied and praise the name of the Lord.
>
> —Joel 2:25–26 (KJV)

Mrs. Whitman, a health care professional, has testified to the fact that God restores. For years, she said, the enemy had stolen her joy and peace. Nonetheless, after much prayer by her church and family, she discovered that God truly loves and cares for her.

This professional decided to surrender her life to Jesus. Daily personal devotions, Bible reading, and fellowshipping with other Christians are part of her daily walk with God. She is giving God all the praise, honor, and glory, for He is worthy to be praised. "God restores," she proclaims.

The apostle Paul asserts in Ephesians 3:20 (NKJV), "Now to Him who is able to do exceedingly abundantly above all that we ask or think, according to the power that works in us."

You may be experiencing a time of drought, but this is only for a season. God promises that you will eat and be full and praise His name.

We live in a sinful world, and things happen that could cast doubts. You may have lost someone or something very dear to you, but be assured that the Lord sees and knows everything about you.

However, be confident that the Lord gives power to the faint, and to those who have no might, He increases their strength. Wait on the Lord, and He will renew your strength; you shall mount up with wings like eagles, you will run and not be weary, you will walk and not faint.

A Prayer for Today: Heavenly Father, thank You for restoring the years that the cankerworm has eaten. Your Word is inerrant, and Your promises are true. I love You and adore You. Amen.

Health Nugget: Always remember to eat a well-balanced diet, with six servings of fruits and vegetables every day. If you are diabetic or have cardiac or kidney disease, adhere to your prescribed diet. Get regular checkups with your primary care physician, and see specialists as warranted.

Hope and Prosperity Gem: Blessed are the pure in heart, for they will see the Lord. Abundance and prosperity are yours for the asking if you keep God at the center of your life. He promises to give you the desires of your heart.

I Will Restore the Years of Plenty

The years that the locusts have eaten,
I will restore.
All the precious moments they have taken,
I will give you even more.

The locusts may have torn your life apart;
they may have cause disarray.
But your troubles will soon depart,
for Jesus will light your way.

God Will Restore

God will restore the years the swarming locust,
the crawling locust, the consuming locust,
and the chewing locust have eaten.
You'll eat in plenty and not be beaten.

Praise the name of the Lord our God,
for He has done wonderful things.
Praise Him in the morning and in the evening.
Praise Him and keep on trusting and believing.

God has dealt wonderfully with you
and never will put His people to shame.
Know that the Lord is always with you.
He is the Lord, our God, for there's no other.

Restoration of Stolen Years

Don't be afraid of the years the cankerworm has stolen,
"I, Your God and Father, will restore seven-fold."
Don't worry, for those years of prosperity will be swollen.
For you, He'll continually fashion and mold.

Don't look at the prosperity of the wicked at their door,
for riches gotten unjustly will surely come to naught.
He shall gather them but God will give it
to the righteous and the poor.
So do good and share your wealth, as you ought.

Hell and destruction are never full.
The eyes of man are never satisfied.
Riches do not last forever, not even a pocketful,
some scandalize and tell lies.

The years that the canker worm has eaten will be restored.
So walk in love within and without and fear not.
Yes, said the Lord of Host, the years will be restored.
Trust Him always, and never give up, for He's given you a lot.

Day 13

Unfair Treatment

Teach my Thy way, O Lord, and lead me in a plain path, because of my enemies."

—Psalm 27:11 (KJV)

Do not expect to be treated fairly in this life. People will say and do hurtful things to you, things that you don't deserve. When someone mistreats you, try to use it as an opportunity to grow in grace. See how quickly you can forgive the one who hurts you.

Psalm 37:5–8…11 (KJV) states, "Commit thy way unto the Lord; trust also in him; and he shall bring it to pass. And he shall bring forth thy righteousness as the light, and thy judgment as the noonday. Rest in the Lord, and wait patiently for him: fret not thyself because of him who prospereth in his way, because of the man who bringeth wicked devices to pass. Cease from anger, and forsake wrath: fret not thyself in any wise to do evil. But the meek shall inherit the earth; and shall delight themselves in the abundance of peace."

"The joy of the Lord is your strength," declares Nehemiah 8:10 (NIV). You have nothing to fear. The Lord, our God, is with you and promises that He will never leave you or forsake you. Therefore, you can confidently say that the Lord is my Helper; what can anyone do unto you? They can do nothing to God's children, only what He allows and nothing more. Remember to fight your battles on your knees; pray and seek God.

When you experience an uncertainty in the workplace, remember the Lord says, "Fear thou not; for I am with thee: be not dismayed; for I am thy God: I will strengthen thee; yea, I will help thee; yea, I will uphold thee with the right hand of my righteousness" (Isaiah 41:10 KJV). Even amid unfair treatment, cling to the Lord, and He will fight your battles. Remember, God's outstretched arms embrace you.

A Prayer for Today: Dear Heavenly Father, please help me to forgive and love those who have hurt and wounded me. I choose to forgive them as You have forgiven me. Help me to be a stalwart in the service of the Lord. Amen.

Health Nugget: Drink eight glasses of water, more as needed, especially during the hot summer months. If you are on a fluid-restricted diet, follow your doctor's orders.

Hope and Prosperity Gem: Choose to love and forgive those who mistreat you. God is love.

Unbroken Spirit

Even after brutal inhumane treatment,
the spirit is not broken.
Even in bereavement and grief,
you're still in the process of coping.

How can a fellow human being inflict such pain?
How can our own flesh and blood cause such shame
on their own brother, sister, or child?
We wonder, what do they have to gain?

Is it your sin to blame?
Or is it because you're born in sin and shaped in iniquity?
Should you just hang your head in shame?
You don't have to, for Jesus died on the cross for your liberty.

Be healed and be set free.
Praise God for the victory.
Hallelujah, Amen. Hallelujah, Amen.

It's No Time to Be Afraid

It's no time to be afraid and hide in the forest and glades.
It's no time to cover and retreat.
But it's time to face the foe,
to the battlefront go, with Jesus as your Captain.

Your victory is assured,
Yes, your victory is assured.
Keep fighting the good fight of faith;
Keep Jesus always as your Captain, and you'll win.

With Jesus by your side, you can smile at the storm,
be confident that everything is going to be fine.
For there's no need to worry; you've been reformed.
So go right ahead and throw out your lifeline.

Day 14

Cheerful Countenance

> I have told you this so that my joy may be in you and that your joy may be complete.
>
> —John 15:11 (NIV)

When Christ is the head of your life, He'll give you peace and joy. Your countenance will show it. A cheerful look makes others happy, and good news refreshes the body. Moreover, a happy heart makes a face pleasant, but heartache crushes the spirit. Feed your mind on the Word of God. Spend time daily reading and studying and hiding God's Word in your heart. A person with a cheerful heart has a continual feast.

When the storms of life are raging, God will stand by you. When the job situation seems unbearable and intolerable, look up and ask Him to give you the strength and courage to endure. He will never leave or forsake you; He will come through for you.

No good thing will God withhold from them who walk uprightly. Let your conscience be your guide. Keep your cool. Proverbs 14 and 15 admonish us to have a tranquil and peaceful heart that gives life to the body, but envy makes the bones rot.

Moreover, a soft answer turns away wrath, but a harsh word stirs up anger. And a gentle tongue is a tree of life, but perverseness breaks the spirit. Even so, a glad heart makes a cheerful spirit, and he who is slow to anger quiets contention.

When you reverence the Lord, He'll give you a joyful heart and a happy face. The Lord inhabits the praises of His people. So praise and glorify His Holy name, for He is worthy to be praised.

A Prayer for Today: Heavenly Father, please help me to have a cheerful countenance. Your joy will give me the strength to serve You in spirit and truth. Help me to be faithful to You and to love my neighbor as myself.

Health Nugget: Learn to take life as it comes. Rest in the arms of God, and give your frustrations to Him. Be joyful, and sing the songs of Zion.

Hope and Prosperity Gem: Do not worry or fret. Hold on to Jesus, for He is holding on to you. Victory is yours today. A cheerful countenance is invaluable and the result of a merry heart. Rejoice in the Lord always.

Happiness

Happiness will fill your heart and soul.
Happiness will envelop you throughout.
Happiness will help you climb the pole.
And happiness will cause you to shout.

The goodness of God leads to repentance,
so cast all your cares at His feet.
The goodness of God will make you dance.
Rejoice in the Holy Spirit, for He's so sweet.

Don't Complain

Don't complain when the going gets tough.
Don't complain when the road gets rough.
Don't complain that your cross is heavy.
And don't complain but be grateful and happy.

Changed

Changed within,
changed without.
Changed.
Changed.

I've been changed.
I've been sanctified.
I've been baptized.
I've been changed.

Happy I am,
for I've been changed.
I'll tell you all I can,
for I've been changed.

I've been changed
by the Blood of the Spotless Lamb.
I've been changed.
Oh, how happy I am.

Day 15

Treat Everyone Fairly

> You shall surely give to him, and your heart should not be grieved when you give to him, because for this thing the Lord your God will bless you in all your works and in all to which you put your hand. For the poor will never cease from the land; therefore, I command you, saying, you shall open your hand wide to your brother, to your poor and your needy in your land.
>
> —Deuteronomy 15:10–11 (KJV)

The poor will always be on earth. Treat them well. The Lord says in Matthew 25:35-36 (NIV), "For I was hungry and you gave me something to eat, I was thirsty and you gave me something to drink, I was a stranger and you invited me in, I needed clothes and you clothed me, I was sick and you looked after me, I was in prison and you came to visit me." Do we discriminate between the rich and poor in the method of treatment? Do we treat the rich better than the poor and look at the poor with disdain? We are all brothers and sisters of one bloodline of all nations. Let us love and treat everyone fairly.

God encourages us to treat everyone equally. We live in a fallen world, but with Jesus as the captain and guide in our lives, we can make a difference. As we look around in the workplace or the streets, we can choose to ignore the problems that plague our society, or we could help when the needs arise. Are we self-serving? Or are we willing to get out of our comfort zone and help the poor and needy?

Health care personnel and caregivers have the opportunity to bring hope and goodwill to many of their clients and families. Just a kind word and a compassionate, outstretched arm to embrace the unlovable and untouchable can change a life. Even a genuine smile can make or break a fragile spirit. Our responsibility is great. Therefore, God expects us to lend a helping hand to those in need. We are not working for men but God. So whatsoever we do, let's do it all to the glory of God.

Always follow the golden rule in Luke 6:31 (KJV): "And as ye would that men should do you, do ye also to them likewise." Shun the wrong, and do the right.

A Prayer for Today: Dear Heavenly Father, please help me always to remember the poor and to open my hands to them. Help me to clothe the naked, feed the hungry, provide shelter for the homeless, and always treat everyone with love and compassion, in the name of Jesus, I pray. Amen.

Health Nugget: Soak in the sunshine of God's love. Sunlight is said to give you vitamin D, which helps with vitamin C absorption. Visit your doctor and check your vitamin D level as needed. Use sunscreen as indicated.

Hope and Prosperity Gem: To be prosperous and receive God's most abundant blessings, we must treat others well. We are our brother's keeper.

Tears Should Flow Freely

Tears should flow freely as you think about
the unfair and prejudicial treatment of so many.
Tears should flow freely as you think about
the injustice and the unkindness you experience, if any.

Tears should flow freely as you reminisce.
Tears for what? Tears when you sat by the bench?
Yes, tears for all that has gone wrong.
The tears as you sing your heartfelt song.

How can you and I let the tears flow?
How can you? How can I?
Oh, how I long for the tears to glow,
glistening, glistening down to your toes.

Cleansing tears of repentance, tears of joy;
so leave the tears of sorrow and sweet tranquility enjoy.
If you still have tears that won't cease,
go to Jesus, and He will dry your tears and give you peace.

The Battle Is Real

The harder I try to be nice and kind,
the more resistance I get from every side.
The more loving the words I speak,
the harder the frustrations leak.

As a born-again Christian,
I've often been misunderstood for my devotion.
Nevertheless, I keep praying and believing,
for I know that the Lord promises hope and healing.

The battle for your mind is real,
the constant decisions, the appeal:
"Come to the water of life and drink freely.
for the battle for your mind is real," believe me.

You cannot win this battle all by yourself
because it may cause you to be on a shelf.
Let go of animosity and let God clean you up.
Up, up, up you'll go to Jesus' heavenly sup.

Keep on believing, keep on trusting, no matter how you feel.
For the battle for your mind God can heal.
Keep on praying, keep on loving,
keep on hoping, and keep on forgiving.

Day 16

Cry Out to Jesus

> I cried unto God with my voice, even unto God with my voice; and he gave ear unto me.
>
> —Psalm 77:1 (KJV)

Whenever you are feeling overwhelmed, cry out, "Jesus, help me. Help me, Jesus. Lord, save me." In Matthew 14:19–23 (NKJV), Jesus fed five thousand hungry men, beside women and children, after He prayed and blessed the five loaves and two fish. Immediately Jesus made His disciples get into the boat and go before Him to the other side, while He sent the multitudes away. And when He had sent the multitudes away, He went up on the mountain by Himself to pray.

> Now when evening came, He was alone there. But the boat was now in the middle of the sea, tossed by the waves, for the wind was contrary. Now in the fourth watch of the night Jesus went to them, walking on the sea. And when the disciples saw Him walking on the sea, they were troubled, saying,

"It is a ghost!" And they cried out for fear. But immediately Jesus spoke to them, saying, "Be of good cheer! It is I; do not be afraid." And Peter answered Him and said, "Lord, if it is You, command me to come to You on the water." So He said, "Come." And when Peter had come down out of the boat, he walked on the water to go to Jesus. But when he saw that the wind *was* boisterous, he was afraid; and beginning to sink he cried out, saying, "Lord, save me!" (Matthew 14:24–30 NKJV).

Jesus, in His love and mercy, stretched forth His hand and caught him. This same Jesus will do the same for us. If you feel that you are about to sink under the pressures of life and the many decisions you make, call out to Jesus, as Peter did.

The name of the Lord is a strong tower; the righteous run to Him, and He saves them. He is there with His outstretched arms of love and compassion to hold and comfort you. God said to Peter, "'O thou of little faith, wherefore didst thou doubt?' And when they were come into the ship, the wind ceased" (Matthew 14:31-32 KJV).

Just as Jesus immediately helped Peter when he cried out for help, He will do the same for you. He is there with you every step of the way. His love and care for you are real and genuine.

You must tell the Lord all your troubles, for He loves you with an everlasting love. Psychiatrists and counselors can help, but their assistance is limited. Jesus is the only One Who can heal your sin-sick soul. God hears and answers the prayers of a broken and contrite heart.

A Prayer for Today: Dear Heavenly Father, I cry out to You today to save me in this hour of testing and trial; help me to walk in love, faith, hope, and victory. Thank You for hearing and answering my prayer in the name of Jesus. Amen.

Health Nugget: Take time out of your busy schedule to kneel and pray and surrender your life to Jesus. Relax in His presence, and enjoy peace and comfort.

Hope and Prosperity Gem: The Lord promises that no good thing will He withhold from them who walk uprightly. You'll succeed in all areas of your life when you cast all your cares on the Lord.

Don't Lose Hope; Don't Give Up

When you feel so all alone,
with no friends to call your own,
remember Jesus cares and understands.
He'll guide you through the deserted lands.

When you feel that all hope is gone,
remember God is always by your side.
Jesus cares and understands
and with you He will abide.

When you feel like giving up,
remember God has the cup,
the cup of healing and deliverance,
for He knows your circumstance.

Don't lose hope but cry out to Jesus.
He'll rescue you and help you cope, for we're dust.
Yes, Jesus will rescue you, for He's Jesus, our King.
So let's shout praises and sing to Him.

Day 17

God's Workmanship

> For we are God's handiwork, created in Christ Jesus to do good works, which God prepared in advance for us to do.
>
> —Ephesians 2:10 (NIV)

You were made to serve the Lord. The work that you do as a health care worker or caregiver is good. The lives that you touch daily have eternal value.

According to Isaiah, the prophet, "The Spirit of the Lord God is upon me; because the Lord hath anointed me to preach good tidings unto the meek; he hath sent me to bind up the brokenhearted, to proclaim liberty to the captives, and the opening of the prison to them that are bound" (Isaiah 61:1 KJV).

Only what you do for Christ will last; none of the other things you do have eternal value. Taking care of your clients and significant others, giving a kind word, and doing an honest day's work will be rewarded. Don't be discouraged, but remember to continue to do good.

You may be a retired doctor, nurse, chaplain, pastor, nursing aide, physical therapist, occupational therapist, speech therapist, respiratory therapist, mental health counselor, radiologist, and the like, but you can make a difference in the lives of many. All your years of health care experience can be an asset to the younger generation. You could be a consultant or a volunteer. Only as you help others can you help yourself and have a full and abundant life. Share your expertise with others as the opportunity arises.

Besides, 1 Corinthians 15:58 (KJV) declares, "Therefore, my beloved brethren, be ye steadfast, unmovable, always abounding in the work of the Lord, forasmuch as ye know that your labour is not in vain in the Lord."

A Prayer for Today: Dear Father in heaven, thank You for the opportunity to care for my clients; help me to do an honest day's work and always do the very best I can. Please help me to magnify and glorify Your Holy name in all I do and say. Amen.

Health Nugget: Be temperate or moderate in all things. Moderation is the key to health and happiness.

Hope and Prosperity Gem: Continue to fight the good fight of faith, and look to Jesus and live. You are greatly loved.

We Are God's Workmanship

We are God's workmanship, and He has
made provision for us to be saved.
We have no excuse, yes, no excuse;
the price has already been paid, by Jesus whom God raised.
The sacrifice of His life on Calvary's Cross, that's the Good News.

You may not understand the dynamics.
You may not comprehend what's occurring.
You may not believe the complexity of the spiritual warfare,
for the battle for your soul's recurring.

If you only take a look by faith,
you'll see and experience the results on the battle front.
Your spiritual eyes will see the drama,
as you accept Christ and let Him be your forefront.

Your Hands Are Leading Me, Dear Lord

Your hands are leading me
to valleys deep and wide.
Your eyes are directing me,
for in Your presence, I can touch the sky.

My feet will go where You want me to go, dear Lord.
My hands will serve where You want me to serve, dear Lord.
My eyes will look where You want me to look, dear Lord.
My tongue will speak what You want me to say, dear Lord.

So I'll be obedient and go where You want me to go, Lord.
I'm determined to be what You want me to be, Lord.
I'll sing what you want me to sing, Lord.
And I'll preach what You want me to preach, Lord.

A vessel of honor for You, Lord,
a vessel of honor for You.
Mold me and make me into a vessel of honor,
to be Your servant brave and true.

Day 18

Take Care of Yourself

Or do you not know that your body is the Temple of the Holy Spirit who is in you, whom you have from God, and you are not your own?

—1 Corinthians 6:12 (NKJV)

"For ye are bought with a price: therefore glorify God in your body, and in your spirit, which are God's" (1 Corinthians 6:20 KJV). "Whether therefore ye eat, or drink, or whatsoever ye do, do all to the glory of God" (1 Corinthians 10:31 KJV).

Ms. Sylvanie, a hard-working caregiver, worked for several years, taking care of her loved one, without taking a vacation. When asked why she hadn't taken a leave, she said there was no one to relieve her of her duties. Someone in her church suggested she ask someone in her prayer group, but she failed to follow through.

Day after day, night after night, year after year, Ms. Sylvanie continued with that relentless and tedious schedule. Eventually, her body began to break down. First, she started to complain of sleepless nights and headaches, then, dizziness, and frequent urination. These symptoms prompted her to visit her primary care physician. After several diagnostic tests, Ms. Sylvanie was diagnosed with hypertension and type 1 diabetes.

Ms. Sylvanie diligently took her prescribed medications and followed the advice of her doctor. She placed her loved one in a nursing agency. Since that time, Ms. Sylvanie started to take care of herself, and her blood sugar and blood pressure are now under control.

By being in tune with your body and taking care of it, you can experience balance and health. Here are some tips to help you look after your body: have an appropriate balance between work and rest, which will help your body to function well. However, lack of sleep can cause stress and break down your immune system.

God helps those who help themselves. Ms. Sylvanie sought and received help from her doctor. It is imperative to make time in your busy schedule to take care of yourself. Doing this could help you live a long and healthy, productive life.

A Prayer for Today: Dear Heavenly Father, please help me to take excellent care of my body, which is the temple of the Holy Spirit. Thank You for helping me to cast all my cares on You, for You care for me. Amen.

Health Nugget: Vitamin B12 is an important nutrient that supports your cardiovascular system, nervous system, and metabolism.

Hope and Prosperity Gem: Give your burdens to the Lord, and leave them there. Put your trust and confidence in the Lord. He promises to take care of you and abundantly bless the works of your hands.

God Will Take Care of You

God will take care of you,
so give all your problems to Him.
God will take care of you,
so that your light won't go dim.

God will take care of your discouragement.
He will take care of your heartache.
God will take care of your disappointment;
He promises to hold you in His embrace.

He will see you through the darkest night,
and He will take care of you.
Even when no one is in sight,
He's God Almighty, and His steadfast love is true.

God Is for You

If God is for you, who can be against you?
They may ridicule and scandalize your name,
for in God you trust and serve only Thee,
but He loves you just the same.

His own Son God spared not,
for He loved me so much
that He died in my place
and applied His healing touch.

God will fight all your battles,
if you let Him have pre-eminence.
He'll even take care of the herd and cattle,
and pour out His blessings from His omnipotence.

Day 19

Behave Like a Christian

Let love be without dissimulation. Abhor that which is evil; cleave to that which is good. Be kindly affectioned one to another with brotherly love; in honour preferring one another.

—Romans 12:9–10 (KJV)

Behave like a Christian, not only at home or at church but also in the workplace and with friends. Romans 12:10–13 (KJV) states, "Be kindly affectioned one to another with brotherly love; in honour preferring one another; not slothful in business; fervent in spirit; serving the Lord; rejoicing in hope; patient in tribulation; continuing instant in prayer; distributing to the necessity of saints; given to hospitality." You should respect and love everyone. You may not like their attitudes or demeanor but love them anyway, as you love yourself.

Romans 12:14–16 (KJV) declares, "Bless them which persecute you: bless, and curse not. Rejoice with them that do rejoice, and weep with them that weep. Be of the same mind one toward another. Mind not high things, but condescend to men of low estate. Be not wise in your own conceits."

No matter where you are, God is with you. You are never alone.

So go right ahead and live the Christian life. The Lord continues to admonish us not to judge one another about food, drink, or holy days, for all will stand before the judgment seat of God.

Love everyone, even the pessimists. Behaving like a Christian necessitates that you adhere to the requirements of God, as stated in Micah 6:6–8 (KJV): "He hath shewed thee, O man, what is good; and what doth the LORD require of thee, but to do justly, and to love mercy, and to walk humbly with thy God?" Therefore, always do the right thing, be quick to forgive, harbor no ill-will or hatred toward anyone, and humble yourself before the mighty hand of God.

A person who walks in pride will be humbled. As you endeavor to keep these requirements with the help of the Holy Spirit, you'll indeed be a conduit in which the Holy Ghost dwells.

"In the same way, let your light shine before others, that they may see your good deeds and glorify your Father in heaven" (Matthew 5:16 NIV). As you put Jesus first and foremost in your life, the world will see Jesus in and through you. Don't hide your light under a bushel, but put it on a lampstand for all to see.

With Christ as the center of your life, you will exude confidence, and the fruit of the Spirit will be apparent in your life. For that reason, don't be afraid to tell the world about God's love. Therefore, be a brave soldier in the army of the Lord, and fight the good fight of faith. Be strong and courageous.

A Prayer for Today: Dear Heavenly Father, please help me not to cause anyone to stumble but instead help me to be humble, kind, and meek. Let Your light shine through me for all to see and bring glory to Your Holy name. Amen.

Health Nugget: Vitamin B12 is usually found in animal products such as meat, eggs, and dairy; for total vegetarians and vegans, it can be found in ready-to-eat breakfast cereals and fortified plant beverages like soy, rice, almond, and coconut milk.

Hope and Prosperity Gem: No matter what issues may assail you, remember, God is on your side. You are more than a conqueror to Him Who loves you. The Lord will prosper and give you the desires of your heart when you acknowledge Him in all your ways.

Lord, I Want to Be a Christian

Lord, I want to be a Christian who's honest and true.
Lord, I want to be a soldier for You.
Lord, I want to be a servant like You.
Lord, I want to be a Christian who's true.

Lord, I want to be more like You.
Give me a heart like Thine,
a heart that's tender and true,
that will serve humankind and You.

A genuine servant and nothing less,
a gentle spirit I want to possess,
a generous steward I want to be,
and a merciful Savior You are to me.

You Can Make a Difference

You can make a difference
in a life of compromise.
You can make a difference
by being very precise.

Tell them about Jesus and His love.
Tell them how He suffered
and the Holy Ghost descended as a dove,
and when His disciples were astonished and shuddered.

I'll tell you about Jesus.
Oh, what a difference
He'll make in your life.
Take time for reverence.

You can make a difference
in this sin-cursed earth.
You can make a difference
with your new Christian birth.

You can make a difference.
Yes, you can make a difference.

Day 20

Forgiveness: A Key to Health

Forgive as God has forgiven you.

—Matthew 6:13 (NKJV)

Forgiveness is the key to health and happiness. When you forgive, it frees you to walk in victory and enjoy the abundant blessings of the Lord. If you refuse to forgive and harbor bitterness and resentment in your heart, you are only hurting yourself. Disease and debilitation may be the result. So why not purpose in your heart to let go of grudges, resentment, offenses, and forgive?

You are correct; it's easier said than done. I understand; I've been there too. It took me several years to get a grip on the severity of holding on to grudges and unforgiveness. As a result, I had no peace and joy. Fortunately, I purposed in my heart to forgive and asked the Lord to forgive me as well; joy and peace flooded my soul. Determine in your heart to release those festering emotions that are holding you hostage, and enjoy the peace of God.

The individual you are holding a grudge against is often free and enjoying life. For heaven's sake, let go, and let God change your heart. He is willing and able to do just that.

With genuine sincerity of heart and mind, ask the Lord to help you to forgive, and He will. Leave your bitterness and anger at the foot of the cross, and leave them there. Don't go back and pick them up. God can do for you what no one else can do. He is willing and able to help you and set you free to enjoy life to the fullest. Pray and leave the consequences to Him, for He's a just judge.

For me to gain the victory over anger and resentment, I had to resolve in my heart to forgive as Christ has forgiven me. I even wrote down all the things that caused the problem, then prayed over them, tore up the paper, and then burned them. After I did that, I felt as free as a bird. Peace, joy, hope, and happiness flooded my heart and soul. Praise the Lord; I'm still walking in that freedom. All praise, honor, and glory go to the Lord for His steadfast love and forgiveness.

God admonishes us to "remember ye, not the former things, neither consider the things of old. Behold, I will do a new thing; now it shall spring forth; shall ye not know it? I will even make a way in the wilderness, and rivers in the desert" (Isaiah 43:18-19 KJV).

Letting go of anger and resentment and freely forgiving the perpetrator is liberating. The Lord wants us to be free. He says, "For I know the thoughts that I think toward you, saith the Lord, thoughts of peace, and not of evil, to give you an expected end" (Jeremiah 29:11 KJV).

"O come let us worship and bow down and kneel before the Lord our Maker" (Psalm 95:6 NIV). This posture will help you to forgive and enjoy the key to health and wellness.

A Prayer for Today: Dear Heavenly Father, You are great and awesome. You heal the broken-hearted, set the captives free, and give liberty to them who are bruised and wounded. Thank You for setting me free. Please help me always be willing to forgive as You have forgiven me, so that I can walk in freedom and enjoy peace and blessings, in the name of Jesus. Amen.

Health Nugget: The digestion of vitamin B12 begins in the stomach, where gastric secretions split vitamin B12 from proteins. For efficient absorption, a B12 tablet must be chewed rather than swallowed.

Hope and Prosperity Gem: Only God can unclog the clogged or plugged drain or pipe of your heart due to anger, resentment, hostility, grudge, and unforgiveness. Surrender all to the Lord, and let Him unclog the dictates of your heart so that He can freely pour His love and forgiveness.

Forgiveness

Forgiveness is the final test.
Do you choose to forgive or not?
Forgiveness will give you rest,
so what will be your test?

It's giving up your right to punish,
an eye for an eye and a tooth for a tooth.
No, for that's absolutely outlandish,
rather choose to forgive, even if they loot.

Forgiveness is what you need,
so choose to forgive yourself.
Choose to forgive and take heed
and ask God to heal you Himself.

Come to the altar of forgiveness.
Come where the cleansing river flows.
Come to a place of sweet repose.
Come to the fountain so deep that glows.

Forgive and Forget

If you forgive others the wrongs they've done,
our Heavenly Father will forgive you.
So freely forgive, and the Lord will give you a joyful song.

Choose to forgive and forget,
yes, forget about yesterday's hurt; be happy and don't fret,
for with Jesus you are set, so forgive and forget.

Day 21

Put on the Armor of God

For we wrestle not against flesh and blood, but against principalities, against powers, against the rulers of the darkness of this world, against spiritual wickedness in high places.

—Ephesians 6:12 (KJV)

"Therefore, put on the whole armor of God so that you'll be able to stand in the evil day, and having done all, stand firm. Stand with your belt of truth tight around your waist. Stand therefore, having your loins girt about with truth, and having on the breastplate of righteousness; and your feet shod with the preparation of the gospel of peace; above all, taking the shield of faith, wherewith ye shall be able to quench all the fiery darts of the wicked. And take the helmet of salvation, and the sword of the Spirit, which is the word of God" (Ephesians 6:14–17 KJV).

Always tell the truth, for it will set you free. It's easy to be untruthful, but the results are usually disheartening. Spread the love of God wherever you go, even at work, as the need arises.

"For the word of God is quick, and powerful, and sharper than any two-edged sword, piercing even to the dividing asunder of soul and spirit, and of the joints and marrow, and is a discerner of the thoughts and intents of the heart" (Hebrews 4:12 KJV). Reading, meditating, and obeying the Word of God will help you to defeat the cunning tricks of the devil. Pray without ceasing, and in everything, give thanks to the Lord, for this is His will concerning you.

A Prayer for Today: Dear Lord, please help me always to put on Your armor and keep my eyes on You. Grant me to know Your will and help me to heartily and willing to do it without murmuring or complaining. And Lord, whatever letter You choose to write on my heart, let it be a letter of the fullness of praise to You, in the name of Jesus, I pray. Amen.

Health Nugget: Sugary drinks are said to be very fattening and associated with obesity, type 2 diabetes, heart disease, cancer, and other health problems. Drink water instead.

Hope and Prosperity Gem: As you put on the armor of God and keep it on, He will protect and keep you in health even as your soul prospers. God's favor is on those who trust and faithfully serve Him.

Four Ways to Conquer Temptation

First, refocus your attention on something virtuous and true.
Second, reveal your struggle to a godly friend.
Third, resist the devil, and he will flee from you.
Fourth, realize that you are vulnerable and on God depend.

God Fights My Battles

God is for me, so no one can be against me.
He fights my battles, and He always wins.
So I can securely rest and be what He wants me to be.
He has washed and cleansed me from all my sins.

All Things Work Together for Your Good

All things work together for your good,
for Jesus is the Truth and the Light.
His Words are clear and easily understood.
So let the Holy Spirit illuminate your sight.

Sometimes you may wonder and fret
about all the trials and snares that upset.
They are all in God's plan for you.
Therefore, keep the faith and be true.

Trials come to test you sorely.
Temptations rock the boat severely.
Persecution raises its ugly head,
but "Be encouraged," Jesus said.

The road may be rough,
life may be tough,
but with Jesus, you can safely go,
even in this world of trouble and woe.

Day 22

Materialism's Influence

> And be not conformed to this world: but be ye transformed by the renewing of your mind, that ye may prove what is that good, and acceptable, and perfect, will of God.
>
> —Romans 12:2 (NKJV)

In our society, the things of the world (the glitz, amusements, and shining lights) seem so exciting, but in reality, they're a waste of time.

Materialism is on the rise and one of the maladies of the modern era. The Joneses: Do you want to be like them? What about the thousands of billboards and television advertisements promoting materialism? The more, the better. Many people spend their lives working themselves to the bone, keeping up with the Joneses to the detriment of their health and well-being. Chronic diseases like high blood pressure, heart disease, stroke, cancer, and kidney disorders are rampant and getting worse.

Philippians 4:19 (NKJV) proclaims: "And my God shall supply all your need, according to his riches in glory by Christ Jesus." Likewise, Philippians 4:11-13 (KJV) affirms, "Not that I speak in respect of want: for I have learned, in whatsoever state I am, therewith to be content. I know both how to be abased, and I know how to abound: every where and in all things I am instructed both to be full and to be hungry, both to abound and to suffer. I can do all things through Christ which strengtheneth me."

I've known health care professionals who have had two and three jobs to try to keep up with the Joneses. As a result of overtaxing their bodies, several have succumbed to chronic debilitating diseases, and some have died.

The apostle Paul counsels us in 1 Timothy 6:6–8 (KJV) that "godliness with contentment is great gain. For we brought nothing into this world, and it is certain we can carry nothing out. And having food and raiment let us be therewith content."

Here's my winsome and godly mother's advice: "Eat little and live long." God is faithful and will supply all that you need.

A Prayer for Today: Dear Heavenly Father, even when I'm under pressure, help me to reflect the brightness of Jesus' love, joy, and peace to a dying world. Show me how to be temperate in all things and enjoy the fruits of my labor and not to cause pain, as Jabez prayed, in the name of Jesus. Amen.

Health Nugget: Avoid processed junk foods, for they're deficient in nutrients and vitamins. They have the propensity to make you fat. These foods are high in fat, sugar, and empty calories (micronutrients) and low in fiber and protein.

Hope and Prosperity Gem: The blessing of the Lord makes you productive and adds no anguish to it.

Jabez's Prayer

Jabez prayed so hard and sincerely that his prayer was heard.
Jabez knew that he was conceived in much pain,
yet nothing deterred him from answering the call,
no matter how hard and difficult the fast lane.

Jabez prayed, Lord, please increase my territory,
so that I would not cause pain as before.
Please expand my task as a visionary,
so that I will no longer be fearful and poor.

I'm not asking for riches or fame
but for showers of blessing,
so that I can help those they defame,
the poorest of the poor, I'm confessing.

Jabez, yes, that's my name, a name that means pain.
Pain coming in, pain going out.
But pain will not define me.
Thank you, Lord, Hallelujah, for changing
my name to being one of fame.

Too Much of Anything Is Bad for You

Too much of anything
is bad for you.
Too little of everything
could be bad too.

You can find a perfect balance
in the One Who calms the raging sea;
you can find your perfect stance
in the One Who made you free.

Day 23

The Desires of the Flesh

> For all that is in the world, the lust of the flesh, and the lust of the eyes, and the pride of life, is not of the Father, but is of the world.
>
> —1 John 2:16 (KJV)

"In whom the god of this world hath blinded the minds of them which believe not, lest the light of the glorious gospel of Christ, who is the image of God, should shine unto them" (2 Corinthians 4:4). Satan blinds the minds of those who are enticed with the deeds of the flesh.

The Lord admonishes us in Galatians 5:19–21 (KJV), "Now the works of the flesh are manifest, which are these; Adultery, fornication, uncleanness, lasciviousness, idolatry, witchcraft, hatred, variance, emulations, wrath, strife, seditions, heresies, envyings, murders, drunkenness, revelings, and such like: of the which I tell you before, as I have also told you in time past, that they which do such things shall not inherit the kingdom of God."

The Lord wants us to serve Him and not be seduced by the deeds of the flesh. Instead, surrender your lives to Him and do right, be merciful, and be humble before Him. If you do these things, you will be blessed and enjoy eternal bliss with Christ and the redeemed.

More cautions regarding the deeds of the flesh are as follows in 1 Corinthians 6:9–10 (KJV): "Know ye not that the unrighteous shall not inherit the kingdom of God? Be not deceived: neither fornicators, nor idolaters, nor adulterers, nor effeminate, nor abusers of themselves with mankind, nor thieves, nor covetous, nor drunkards, nor revilers, nor extortioners, shall inherit the kingdom of God."

God desires us to successfully overcome the lures of the flesh and live a holy life. He is our constant help, every step of the way. Lean on Him today and always. The problem is in the flesh due to the Fall of man and sin. "The flesh lusteth against the Spirit, and the Spirit against the flesh: and these are contrary the one to the other: so that ye cannot do the things that ye would" (Philippians 5:17 KJV).

The apostle Paul declares in Romans 8:1, 5–8 (KJV), "There is therefore now no condemnation to them which are in Christ Jesus, who walk not after the flesh, but after the Spirit. For they that are after the flesh do mind the things of the flesh; but they that are after the Spirit the things of the Spirit. For to be carnally minded is death; but to be spiritually minded is life and peace. Because the carnal mind is enmity against God: for it is not subject to the law of God, neither indeed can be. So then they that are in the flesh cannot please God." Thus, God desires us to be holy as He is holy. We can only attain this holiness if we keep our eyes on Him and love Him with all our hearts and love our neighbors as ourselves.

Therefore, let the mind of Christ be in you as you endeavor to do His will, as it pleases Him. He will give you the strength and courage to live for Him. The Lord qualifies and empowers those He calls.

As you walk and talk with the Lord, you'll bear much fruit, the fruit of the Spirit, which is "love, joy, peace, longsuffering, gentleness, goodness, faith, meekness, temperance: against such there is no law" (Galatians 5:22–23 KJV).

The apostle John affirms in 1 John 2:15–17 (KJV), "Love not the world, neither the things that are in the world. If any man love the world, the love of the Father is not in him. For all that is in the world, the lust of the flesh, and the lust of the eyes, and the pride of life, is not of the Father, but is of the world. And the world passeth away, and the lust thereof: but he that doeth the will of God abideth forever."

Lastly, "Therefore if any man be in Christ, he is a new creature: old things are passed away; behold, all things are become new" (2 Corinthians 5:17 KJV). Victory could be yours if you let the Lord help you fight the battle of the flesh.

A Prayer for Today: Dear Heavenly Father, help us to focus on You and not the works of the flesh but of the Spirit. You are God and God alone and well able to deliver us. Help us to be strong in the power of Your might, now and always. Thank You for hearing and answering our prayers, in the name of Jesus. Amen.

Health Nugget: The oil in ginger is a useful herbal remedy for nasal and chest congestion. Ginger is also said to be good for nausea and motion sickness. Ginger makes a delicious tea; use it as needed.

Hope and Prosperity Gem: As you keep your focus on the Lord and His promises and not on the things of the world, you'll discover joy, peace, and prosperity in all areas of your life.

Repentance: A Free Gift

True repentance in Greek is *metanoia,*
which literally means "a change of mind."
True repentance is a far cry from paranoia
and a free gift of the sublime.

Repentance, like faith,
will your sad and depressed spirit lift.
So don't wait until it's too late
to accept salvation as an eternal gift.

The Lord's provision is individually efficacious
for those who accept His death on the cross;
His favor and grace are precious.
For those who accept His gift would not suffer loss.

God Chooses Whom He Would

God uses and chooses things
the world calls foolish.
He calls the lonely, the weak,
the despised, for God they'll seek.

He shames the wise,
He shames the mighty,
so that no flesh
should glory in His presence.

If you feel you're only a nobody,
review God's call to Gideon,
and then you'll realize you're a somebody,
for God wants to use you, like the "just and devout" man, Simeon.

God uses ordinary people to carry out His
extraordinary work and plan,
so that no flesh can glory in His presence.
Here I am, Lord; use me in Your work and in Your plan.
I glory in the cross of shame and bask in Your presence.

Day 24

The Allurement of Riches

> No one can serve two masters. Either you will hate the one and love the other, or you will be devoted to the one and despise the other. You cannot serve both God and money.
>
> —Matthew 6:24 (NKJV)

The allurement of riches is real. Many health care workers and caregivers alike, including born-again Christians, are mesmerized by the fleeting pleasures of sin and the prospect of riches and the good life.

As we keep our eyes on Jesus, the things of the world will grow strangely dim in the light of His glory and grace. The Lord says in 1 Timothy 6:10 (KJV) that "the love of money is the root of all evil: which while some coveted after, they have erred from the faith, and pierced themselves with many sorrows." Turn to Jesus and live. Serve Him wholeheartedly, and He'll give you a life of peace and abundance. As you surrender your heart to the Lord, remember to watch and pray and keep your eyes on Him.

Because of the allurement of riches, wealth, and fame, many Christians have faltered in their faith. Be grateful for the blessings of the Lord, whether they be little or much.

Be content with the blessings of the Lord. Many have lost their lives amassing wealth. So why not be satisfied with what you have? God promises to give you everything you need. "Better is a little with righteousness than great revenues without right" (Proverbs 16:8 KJV).

The trials of this life are many, but with God's help and your unwavering faith in His promises, you can live a victorious and prosperous life. Jesus declares in Isaiah 43:1–2 (KJV), "Fear not, for He has redeemed you, and called you by His Name, for you are His. When you walk through the waters, He will be with you, and through the rivers, they shall not overflow you, when you walk through the fire, you shall not be burned, nor shall the flame scorch you." Believe in the promises of God, and be content.

A Prayer for Today: Dear Heavenly Father, I rejoice in the freedom that the Holy Spirit gives to help me live in the light of Your presence. Help me not to be allured by the accumulation of riches to the detriment of my walk with Thee. Remove anything in my life that would hinder Your blessing, in the name of Jesus. Amen.

Health Nugget: Rubbing peppermint oil, tiger balm, or white flower oil into your temples may reduce tension headaches and some forms of stress. These three remedies contain menthol as well as analgesic properties.

Hope and Prosperity Gem: Turn your eyes upon Jesus and bask in the garden of His love. As you put Him first and foremost in your life, you could experience victory.

Riches Cannot Redeem

Silver and gold,
rubies and diamonds,
pearl and amethyst,
topaz and chrysoprase,

sapphire and emerald,
jasper and chrysolite,
precious stones galore
and beautiful ornaments and much more.

Riches cannot redeem
Only Jesus' blood washes our sins clean.

Eyes Blinded by Riches

Many hearts have become hardened and callous
by the cares of this world.
Their hearts have become cold and malicious,
and their eyes have been blinded by riches untold.

But here am I, Lord, send me.
I'll go where You want me to go.
Here am I, Lord, send me;
I'll be Your eyes not blinded by riches, so I'll go.

Day 25

Filling Your Barns

> And Jesus said to them, "Take heed and beware of covetousness: for a man's life consisteth not in the abundance of the things he possesseth."
>
> —Luke 12:15 (KJV)

Filling your barns with plenty is something that many people desire. In the parable of the rich man as told by Jesus in Luke 12:19–21 (KJV), a young man did just that. He planned to sit down in ease and enjoy life. That same night would have been his last. His plans were to break down his existing barns and build bigger and better ones, eat, drink, and be merry for many years. "But God said to him, 'Fool! This night your soul will be required of you; then whose will those things be which you have provided?' So is he who lays up treasure for himself, and is not rich toward God."

This rich fool was concerned about himself. Filling your storehouses with more and more things is one of the cunning tricks and snares of the devil. Many Christians, including health care personnel, are more concerned about filling their homes with trinkets, silver, and gold. Beware. The enemy is cunning and full of tricks.

The parable of the rich fool is widespread today. Many have

laid up treasures for themselves and are not rich toward God, the Provider of all things. At the end, who would inherit all your possessions? The person who inherits your properties may squander them and have no regard for the sweat and tears that went into amassing those possessions.

In Matthew 19:21–24 (KJV), Jesus said unto the councilman, "'If thou wilt be perfect, go and sell that thou hast, and give to the poor, and thou shalt have treasure in heaven: and come and follow me.' But when the young man heard that saying, he went away sorrowful: for he had great possessions. Then said Jesus unto his disciples, 'Verily I say unto you, that a rich man shall hardly enter into the kingdom of heaven. And again, I say unto you, it is easier for a camel to go through the eye of a needle, than for a rich man to enter into the kingdom of God.'" Give your all to Jesus, and He will abundantly bless you and your household.

A Prayer for Today: Dear Heavenly Father, thank You for Your many blessings that You've given us to enjoy. Help us to be rich toward You and store up our treasures in heaven, where moth and rust cannot destroy and where thieves cannot break through and steal, in the name of Jesus. Amen.

Health Nugget: Invest in a good pair of sneakers, and enjoy a brisk walk daily. Physical activity will help to increase your energy level, especially if you are fighting fatigue and lethargy. Drink an adequate amount of water to keep hydrated.

Hope and Prosperity Gem: Where your treasure is, your heart longs to be there. Thus, "lay up for yourselves treasures in heaven, where neither moth nor rust doth corrupt, and where thieves do not break through nor steal" (Matthew 6:20 KJV).

Wide or Narrow Road

What road will you be finding?
The broad and wide, or the narrow and winding?
The broad and wide road may lead to annihilation.
So choose the narrow and winding road, which
leads to eternal bliss and sin eradication.

Again, the straight and broad way leads to death and destruction,
while the narrow and winding way leads to life and liberation.
I choose to walk the narrow road,
with all its trials and heavy load.
I choose to persevere under strife;
I choose Jesus Christ.

The People Sat Down to Play

The people sat down and then rose up to play.
Oh, it's going to be a brighter day.
They say it's going to be a brighter day,
for the end of time is far away.

The end of time is far away,
so why should we worry or pray?
Let's continue to marry and divorce,
for we have lots of resource.

Don't you ever fool yourselves,
Jesus is waiting right at the door.
He's gently knocking as your heart melts,
so let Him in, for your sins He bore.

Day 26

Christian Living

> There shall not any man be able to stand before thee all the days of thy life: as I was with Moses, so I will be with thee: I will not fail thee, nor forsake thee. Be strong and of a good courage: for unto this people shalt thou divide for an inheritance the land, which I sware unto their fathers to give them.
>
> —Joshua 1:5–6 (KJV)

No matter where you are, God is with you. You are never alone. Health care workers and caregivers, you can and should maintain your Christian witness, whether you are caring for a belligerent client or a gentle one. Do not leave your Christianity at the door but always take it with you, for the Lord promises that He will be with you wherever you go.

Several years ago, when I was thumbing through some papers under my bed, I found the verse above; I've held on to it ever since. The Lord has been my constant Companion and Friend, who has been holding my right hand with His victorious right hand. I have nothing to fear, for my God is always with me.

He often reminds me to be strong and courageous, for the battle is not mine but His. Here's another scripture that has given me strength and courage for the journey: "For God hath not given us the spirit of fear; but of power, and of love, and of a sound mind" (2 Timothy 1:7 KJV).

Let's encourage one another in love. No matter what issues may assail you, remember that God is on your side. You are more than a conqueror through Him Who loves you and died for you. There is no greater love than Jesus' love for you. Embrace God's love, and He'll help you to live a victorious Christian life.

A Prayer for Today: Dear Heavenly Father, I look to You for direction and guidance. Help me to be strong and courageous, for You're an ever-present help in the time of trouble. Help me to live the Christian life wherever I go, in the name of Jesus. Amen.

Health Nugget: According to some research, a whiff of the aromatic herb rosemary may increase alertness and improve memory.

Hope and Prosperity Gem: As we endeavor to live the Christian life, God promises us that if we call upon Him with sincerity of heart, mind, and spirit, He will prosper us and give us a glorious future.

Be Strong and of Good Courage

God said, "Just as I was with Moses,
I'll be with you.
Be strong and of good courage,
For I'm right there with you.

Don't look to the right.
Don't look to the left.
Don't look at man's eyes,
for they could be deceiving sights.

"I've called you in such a time as this.
I'm sheltering you under the shadow of My wings.
I'm guiding your footsteps,
for I've called you to do great things.

Be strong and courageous,
for I'm with you."
Joshua 1 (KJV)

Take Time to Be Holy

Take time to be holy.
Take time to service render.
Take time to praise Jesus.
Take time to surrender.

Take time to ponder.
Take time to remember God's goodness.
Take time to serve your fellow men.
Take time to bask in His lovingkindness.

Take time for family.
Take time for friends.
Take time to love and pray
and receive the gift of salvation today.

Day 27

Be Not Afraid

Fear thou not; for I am with thee. Be not dismayed; for I am thy God: I will strengthen thee; yea, I will help thee; yea, I will uphold thee with the right hand of My righteousness.

—Isaiah 41:10 (KJV)

"And the LORD, He it is that doth go before thee; He will be with thee, he will not fail thee, neither forsake thee: fear not, neither be dismayed" (Deuteronomy 31:8 KJV). Remember to take one day at a time, and God will give you the strength and courage you need. His Word is true, and His promises are true. Jesus declares "I am the way, the truth, and the life: no man cometh unto the Father, but by Me" (John 14:6 KJV).

No struggle, no growth. Therefore, in order to not be afraid, give all your concerns and problems to Jesus. Remember: the way the

Lord has led you in the past should remind you of His faithfulness and love.

Do not be afraid because in being fearful, you can torment yourself. The Lord is faithful to all His promises and has remembered you in His love and mercy. God has poured out His grace upon you so you can share His love and goodness with others.

God will never give you more than you can handle, and He will help you get through difficult times. After He does, you'll be able to look back and smile, and realize that you made it through the storm. God promises that He will never leave you nor forsake you.

The Lord is on your side; you are the apple of His eye. Luke 12:7 (KJV) declares, "But even the very hairs of your head are all numbered. Fear not therefore: ye are of more value than many sparrows." God loves you so much that He watches over you every minute of every day. The Lord says to you in Isaiah 49:16 (KJV), "Behold, I have graven thee upon the palms of My hands; thy walls are continually before Me."

Hold on to Jesus, for He is always by your side. No other friend in this world loves and cares for you like Jesus. Did you know that He is closer than the very breath you breathe? So don't be afraid of the dark, for Jesus is with you.

The same God who protected Elisha from his enemies is the very same God who's protecting you. So why are you afraid of the enemy? The Lord says emphatically that He will take care of you. Lay all your burdens, fears, frustrations, and anxieties at the foot of the cross and leave them there. God is a God of impossibilities.

Jeremiah 32:27 (KJV) affirms, "Ah Lord God! behold, Thou hast made the heaven and the earth by Thy unlimited power and outstretched arm, and there is nothing too hard for Thee." He fights your battles for you. The Lord God Almighty wants you to have faith and confidence in Him.

Here are two scriptures to help you find peace for your troubled soul: First, Jesus said, "Peace I leave with you, my peace I give unto you: not as the world giveth, give I unto you. Let not your heart be troubled, neither let it be afraid" (John 14:27 KJV). Second, the psalmist David declares, "Yea, though I walk through the valley of the shadow of death, I will fear no evil: for thou art with me; thy rod and thy staff they comfort me" (Psalm 23:4 KJV).

You don't have to be afraid; just put your trust and confidence in God, who loves you with an everlasting love. His love is steadfast, genuine, more profound than the deepest ocean, more extensive than the broadest sea, and higher than the highest mountain. That's God's love for you.

A Prayer for Today: Dear Heavenly Father, thank You for Your precious promises; we don't have to fear, for You're right there to fight our battles, in the name of Jesus. Amen.

Health Nugget: To help ease anxiety and stress, and get a good night's sleep, soak in a hot tub with a few drops of lavender essential oil. Listen to your favorite soothing music to unwind further.

Hope and Prosperity Gem: Do not be afraid, for God is with you and will never leave you nor forsake you. The Lord also promises to bless you if you obey His commandments.

Don't Be Afraid of the Dark

Don't be afraid of the dark,
for Jesus has set your mark.
Don't sit and be still.
Work and work until.

Don't be afraid of the dark,
for God's light shines bright
all around the world.
Yes, His light is shining all around the world.

Don't lose hope, my friend.
Don't lose hope;
Jesus is close to your side.
With you, He will abide.

Face Your Fear

Face fear. Face fear. Face fear.
Get up and do what you fear the most.
Do it with ado and gusto.
Do what you fear to do the most.

Deliverance can be yours,
so just trust and lean on the Lord.
Don't look and fan your fear,
but run to Jesus and read and obey His Word.

The Lord has not given you a spirit of fear
but of power, and of love, and of a sound mind.
So come on, be strong and of good courage and cheer.
Believe in your heart, and then joy and peace you'll find.

Day 28

Hope in God

> "For I know the plans I have for you," says the Lord, "plans for well-being and not for trouble, to give you a future and a hope."
>
> —Jeremiah 29:11 (NIV)

We have a sure and steadfast anchor of the soul. Romans 8:38–39 (KJV) states that "neither death, nor life, nor angels, nor principalities, nor powers, nor things present, nor things to come, nor height, nor depth, nor any other creature, shall be able to separate us from the love of God, which is in Christ Jesus our Lord."

Furthermore, He longs to give you a bright future with favor, prosperity, and full life, but only if we walk uprightly and obey Him. The apostle Paul affirms in Ephesians 3:20 (KJV), "Now unto Him who is able to do exceedingly abundantly above all that we ask or think, according to the power that worketh in us." Will you trust Him today? The Lord loves you with an everlasting love.

Focus your mind on the Lord, and He will give you perfect peace. Moreover, give your plans to God, for He knows where He wants you to go.

The Lord also declares, "And thine ears shall hear a word behind thee, saying, this is the way, walk ye in it, when ye turn to the right hand, and when ye turn to the left" (Isaiah 30:21 KJV). "And the God of peace shall bruise Satan under your feet shortly. The grace of our Lord Jesus Christ be with you. Amen" (Romans 16:20 KJV).

As health care workers and caregivers, the tasks at hand may be overwhelming with nowhere to run and hide, but you can hide in the outstretched arms of God. When you feel all alone, and no one understands your frustration and exhaustion, put your trust and confidence in the Lord. He says that He will never leave you nor forsake you. Psalm 42:11 (KJV) says, "Why art thou cast down, O my soul? And why art thou disquieted within me? Hope thou in God; for I shall praise Him, who is the health of my countenance, and my God."

Because of the high demand and severe shortage of health care workers, many employees have experienced burnout. The burnout rate in health care is extremely high, especially among physicians in training, clinicians, and nurses. Burnout is a syndrome marked with emotional and mental exhaustion that results in decrease accomplishment and effectiveness at work. The heavy workload could lead to fatigue, poor concentration, time constraints, and role conflicts.

During my extensive career as a registered nurse, I experienced the burnout syndrome due to a heavy workload, long hours, and frequent covering of nursing staff shortages. Stress and physical and emotional overexertion triggered migraine headaches, according to my primary care physician. However, I thank the Lord for His goodness, mercy, and grace; I took an extended leave of absence to relax and smell the roses. "The Lord is my portion, saith my soul; therefore will I hope in Him" (Lamentation 3:24 NKJV).

Take frequent mental breaks, likewise, to avoid fatigue and emotional exhaustion. Take one day at a time, and "do not worry about tomorrow, for tomorrow will worry about itself. Each day has enough trouble of its own" (Matthew 6:34 NIV). Take time to rest. Take time to travel and enjoy your family.

Most importantly, take time to know God and read and meditate on His Word. Take one day at a time, and savor every moment. Slow down and relax. God wants you to prosper and be in good health and enjoy the fruit of your labor.

A Prayer for Today: Dear Heavenly Father, help me to remember that my hope and security are in You. Show me any areas of my life that may be hindering faith and hope; help me to overcome, in the name of Jesus. Amen.

Health Nugget: People whose diet is rich in potassium may be less prone to high blood pressure and kidney disease. Reducing sodium intake and eating bananas, cantaloupes, and oranges may help to keep your heart healthy. These fruits are high in potassium.

Hope and Prosperity Gem: "Come to Me, all you who labor and are heavy laden, and I will give you rest" (Matthew 11:28 NKJV). God wants to give you hope and a future full of His wonderful blessings. Just keep Him in the center of all you do and say.

Thank You, Lord, for Hope

My pen and ink cannot express my gratitude
to my Maker and my King,
for He's the One Who gives me latitude
to praise and worship; to Him I sing.

Lord, You are incredible and help me to cope,
for You're touched with the feelings
of my infirmities and have given me hope.
Lord, thank You for helping me with my dealings.

Deep inside the recesses of my mind,
You are there, leading and guiding me.
When no one seems to care when I'll in a bind,
I can feel Your hand in mine.

Lord, You are merciful and kind and sensitive to my pain.
You are the hope of the world.
The King of kings and Lord of lords.
Thank You, Lord, for Your Word, the Sword.

Day 29

You're a Winner

> Do you not know that in a race all the runners run, but only one gets the prize? Run in such a way as to get the prize.
>
> —1 Corinthians 9:24 (NIV)

The apostle Paul reminds us in 1 Corinthians 9:25–27 (KJV), "And every man that striveth for the mastery is temperate in all things. Now they do it to obtain a corruptible crown; but we an incorruptible. I therefore so run, not as uncertainly; so fight I, not as one that beateth the air: But I keep under my body, and bring it into subjection: lest that by any means, when I have preached to others, I myself should be a castaway."

Therefore, let us run to win the prize, eternal life. A certain man started running a marathon and was doing well until he fell; he injured his leg and was forced to drop out of the race. However, another man began the race with a very slow and steady pace. Even though many runners passed him, he successfully finished the race and got a trophy like the others.

The race of life is much the same. Many started out trusting and serving the Lord, but when trials and temptations overwhelmed them, they stopped running the race and returned to their previous life of sin and worldly pleasures. Which one do you think would win the race of life? The one who stopped by the wayside, or the one who endured to the end? Yes, the one who suffered to the end amid the storms of life. That's the same one who will hear, "Well done, thou good and faithful servant." Therefore, as a health care worker, run your race in your lane.

Continue to do good and provide the very best care to all your clients. The Lord will reward you.

A Prayer for Today: Dear Father in heaven, help us to examine ourselves daily and recognize that we are winners because You made us. We are Your people and the sheep of Your pasture. Thank You for valuing us so much that You sent Jesus to die for our sins. John 3:16 (KJV) declares, "For God so loved the world, that he gave his only begotten Son, that whosoever believeth in him should not perish, but have everlasting life."

Health Nugget: Probiotics, good bacteria, are live microorganisms intended to provide health benefits when consumed; they help to improve the flora of the stomach and the gastrointestinal tract (gut).

Hope and Prosperity Gem: You're a winner. A winner never quits. A quitter never wins; even when the going gets tough, hang in there, for the Lord will help you. Hold on to your integrity, for you are a conqueror, indeed.

Is Jesus the Love of Your Life?

Is Jesus the love of your life?
Is Jesus the hope of your joy?
As you trust Him, He'll get sweeter as the days go by.
Keep singing new song, and His blessings you'll enjoy.

He loves you deeply.
He loves you sincerely.
He loves you passionately.
Yes, He loves you unconditionally.

You're lost and undone without Him.
He'll fill you up to the brim,
for your very existence depends on him.
That's why you'd sing the "Jesus Loves Me" hymn.

Is Jesus the love of your life?
Is He the joy of your life?
Is He the song that you sing?
Is He your everything?

Born to Be Free

I was born to be free,
born to be the person I ought to be.
I was born to be free,
for there is no one like me.

Born to be nobody but me.
Born to love;
born to dream and hope;
born to be nobody but me.

I can't be you,
and you can't be me,
so let's be ourselves
and accept each other respectfully.

Day 30

Little Is Much with God

> Whoever can be trusted with very little can also be trusted with much, and whoever is dishonest with very little will also be dishonest with much.
>
> —Luke 16:10 (NIV)

When God blesses you, no one can curse you. His blessings supersede anything or anyone in this world. He gives us good things to enjoy as we put our trust and confidence in Him.

Mr. Wilson was a laborer who worked for minimum wage almost all his life; however, he was able to take care of his family. He stretched the small salary he received exponentially after faithfully returning his tithes plus gave generous offerings. Mr. Wilson even had money left over to help the poor and those in need. The more he gave, the more he received, until he was able to purchase his own home and raise his growing family.

The secret of Mr. Wilson's success comes from Malachi 3:10-11 (KJV): "Bring ye all the tithes into the storehouse, that there may be meat in mine house, and prove me now herewith, saith the Lord of hosts, if I will not open you the windows of heaven, and pour you out a blessing, that there shall not be room enough to receive it. And

I will rebuke the devourer for your sakes, and he shall not destroy the fruits of your ground; neither shall your vine cast her fruit before the time in the field, saith the Lord of hosts." Be faithful to the Lord and continue to do His work, and He will bless you. Health care workers and caregivers, God will continue to bless your honest work.

However, if you're disobedient and fail to return to God that which belongs to Him, your tithes, ten percent of your income, you're robbing Him. Malachi 3:8-9 (KJV) says it well: "Will a man rob God? Yet ye have robbed me. But ye say, wherein have we robbed thee? In tithes and offerings. Ye are cursed with a curse: for ye have robbed me, even this whole nation." Therefore, just as Mr. Wilson returned his faithful tithes and love offerings and received God's blessings, I am encouraging you to do the same, if you have not already done so. "Therefore to him that knoweth to do good, and doeth it not, to him it is sin" (James 4:17 KJV).

"For there is no respect of persons with God" (Romans 2:11 KJV). He loves you just like He loves Mr. Wilson and all of His children, whom He created from the dust of the ground. Don't let the devil fool you by believing his lies, for he has been a liar from the beginning.

James 4:7 (NIV) admonishes us to "submit yourselves, then, to God. Resist the devil and he will flee from you." At just the mention of the name of Jesus, the devil will flee. That is the power of His name. Additionally, Philippians 2:10–12 (KJV) says, "Wherefore God has given Him a Name which is above every name: That at the Name of Jesus, every knee should bow, of things in heaven, and things in earth, and things under the earth; And that every tongue should confess that Jesus Christ is Lord to the glory of God the Father. So "fight the good fight of faith, lay hold of eternal life" (1 Timothy 6:12 KJV).

"For God does not show favoritism" (Romans 2:11 NIV). He loves all the same. The main reason Jesus came to earth was to pay the price of sin, by shedding His precious blood on Calvary's cross. That's why you are the apple of His eye. He loves you so much that if you were the only person on earth, Jesus would have left the portals of heaven to die for you. That's how much He loves you.

A Prayer for Today: Dear Heavenly Father, thank You for multiplying my seeds sown for Your kingdom. Thank You also for supplying all my needs, according to Your riches in glory, by Christ Jesus, our Lord. Amen.

Health Nugget: Get a massage at least once a month, if you so desire. Regular massages may help relieve stress and tension and even reduce painful joints. Massage could also help you to relax.

Hope and Prosperity Gem: Little is plenty if God is in it. You may not have lots of money or earthly wealth, but be assured that if you trust God and endure to the end, you will be saved and have eternal life. A life of bliss, happiness, joy, and peace in the presence of our Lord and His holy angels awaits you.

God Is Faithful

God is faithful, for His mercies are new every morning.
Great is Thy faithfulness, Lord, unto me.
Yes, God is faithful, for His mercies are new every morning.
Great is Thy faithfulness, Lord, unto me.

Your lovingkindness is new every morning,
and Your faithfulness is new every night.
Great is Thy faithfulness, Lord, unto me.
Your lovingkindness and love are out of sight.

Cast Your Bread upon the Water

Cast your bread upon the water,
for you will find it after many days.
Jesus told Peter to cast his net a little further,
for you'll catch fish in different ways.

Cast your cares upon the Master,
for you'll find peace and rest.
Cast your love a little faster,
for you'll receive God's best.

Cast your burdens at the foot of the cross,
for you'll find guidance.
Cast yourself at Jesus' feet and in Him be lost,
for you'll find that little is much with deliverance.

Day 31

Watch and Pray and Beware of Temptations

Watch and pray so that you will not fall into temptation. The spirit is willing, but the flesh is weak.

—Mark 14:38 (NIV)

Ms. Dorsey, a health care professional and an excellent musician, was on fire for the Lord and was often found playing her instrument at home and at church. She used her gifts and talents to glorify the Lord. Many admired her natural abilities and performances. However, as she continued to play and received more accolades and commendations, she became very proud of her accomplishments and slowly drifted away from the faith. Proverbs 16:18 (KJV) says, "Pride goeth before destruction, and a haughty spirit before a fall."

The temptation to sin is everywhere, but it is not a sin until you yield to it. James 1:14–15 (KJV) says, "But every man is tempted, when he is drawn away of his own lust, and enticed. Then when lust hath conceived, it bringeth forth sin: and sin, when it is finished, bringeth forth death."

Week after week, Ms. Dorsey's church attendance dwindled and eventually ceased; her inspirational music was silent. Everyone was saddened and felt a sense of loss. Such a God-given talent was no longer present. Ms. Dorsey followed the allurement of the dazzling lights of the world. She failed to watch and pray.

According to 1 Corinthians 10:12–14 (KJV), "Wherefore let him that thinketh he standeth take heed lest he fall. There hath no temptation taken you but such as is common to man: but God is faithful, who will not suffer you to be tempted above that ye are able; but will with the temptation also make a way to escape, that ye may be able to bear it."

After decades of appearing to enjoy the temporary, fleeting pleasures of sin, Ms. Dorsey still has expressed no desire to return to the Lord Jesus, the Savior of the world. God is gracious and merciful and wishes that all should repent and have everlasting life.

2 Corinthians 6:2 (KJV) says, "Behold, now is the accepted time; behold, now is the day of salvation." However, it's not over until it's over. The hope is that one day, Ms. Dorsey will surrender her life to the Lord before it's too late.

Let's pray for one another, for prayer changes things. Prayer is also the key that unlocks the gates of heaven.

A Prayer for Today: Dear Lord, please help us to watch and pray so that we do not enter into temptation because the spirit is willing, but the flesh is weak. Remove any obstacle that is in the way so we can be victorious over trials and enticements.

Health Nugget: Garlic has antiviral and antibacterial properties, whether eaten raw or slightly cooked. It is said to boost your immune functions. If you're self-conscious of the pungent odor of garlic on your breath, try chewing peppermint gum after eating a tiny piece of ginger, or rinsing your mouth with a strong-smelling mouthwash, or eating an apple or fresh lettuce.

Hope and Prosperity Gem: How can we, as individuals, keep ourselves pure in this dark and sinful world? Is there any hope for sinful humanity? The answer is yes; Jesus is the only hope for humanity to live a victorious life.

Don't Be Caught Off-Guard

Don't be caught off-guard,
for this is your charge.
Temptation comes to all, my dear,
so don't despair when it comes near.

Run for your life if you can,
for on your feet you'll safely land.
Hold on to the good and right,
for this is pleasing in God's sight.

When temptation comes a-knocking at your door,
resist the devil, and he will flee some more.
Keep praying and believing this instance,
and read God's Word for deliverance.

Jesus Will Come Again

Why are you gazing into heaven,
men of Galilee?
This same Jesus who was taken up into heaven
will come again, and His face you'll see.

Why stand ye gazing into heaven?
The clouds of angels hung low.
We are happy and not heavy laden
because Jesus, our peace will bestow.

We shall receive power
after the Holy Ghost falls on us like a shower.
Witnesses shall we be
in Jerusalem, and in Judea, and in all the earth for Thee.

Why stand ye gazing into heaven?
Go back to Jerusalem
and wait for the hour
of the Holy Ghost's power.

Be brave. Jesus saves.
He'll come again, just as He said.

Day 32

Weeping May Endure for a Night

> For His anger is but for a moment; His favor is life; Weeping may endure for a night, But joy comes in the morning.
>
> —Psalm 30:5 (NKJV)

With the loss of a loved one, death seems so final and cold. Cry if you may, for this will help relieve the pain and sadness. During a time of loss, it is essential to go through the grieving process to be able to continue living a productive life. Many people say they've never cried or shown any grief. Could it be because they think it's not the manly thing to do? Or could it be pride in showing their vulnerability or humanity?

Grief and sorrow have no boundaries. Cry if you may, and let the tears freely flow. These cleansing tears will help you heal. A good cry will make you feel better.

Psalm 30:5 (KJV) says, "Weeping endureth for a night, but joy cometh in the morning." After you have cried and have gone through the grieving process, you're more likely to show empathy to the grief-stricken.

Mr. Sabastian, a very loving caregiver, lost his spouse several years ago. He reluctantly admitted that he has never cried or gone through the grieving process. As a result, he is still having a difficult time moving forward with his life. There is hope and healing, however, for Mr. Sebastian, if he asks the Lord to help him and seeks professional counseling as needed.

Even during grief, you can cry out to God and give Him praise. He will comfort and hold you in His loving arms. Moreover, God inhabits the praises of His people in the time of loss. Spend time reading and studying God's Word so you can be a tower of strength for those in need.

Even in the workplace, when patients and families lose loved ones and friends, you as a health care worker or caregiver can encourage them and provide supportive care. You can also fortify your mind and spirit with the power of the Holy Spirit and be a beacon of light for the bereaved.

Jesus understands the human heart; He is patient and long-suffering and wishes that none should perish but all should come to repentance and enjoy peace. "For God sent not his Son into the world to condemn the world; but that the world through him might be saved" (John 3:17 KJV).

A Prayer for Today: Dear loving God, please help us to be a source of strength and encouragement to those who've lost loved ones. Help us to show sympathy and empathy and the love of Jesus. Show us how to comfort Your people with loving words. You promised that You would help us and give us no more than we can bear. Thank You, Lord, for Your precious promises. Amen.

Health Nugget: Some other ways to mask or get rid of the odor of garlic and onion on your breath are as follows: use a tongue scraper, brush, and floss, drink water after meals to wash garlic or onion remnants from your tongue and between your teeth.

Hope and Prosperity Gem: You can have peace and enjoy the abundant, victorious life as you look through the lens of hope, faith, and love. Trust and obey God as He leads and guides you into all truth.

You Can Run to Jesus

You can run to Jesus anytime, morning, noon, or night,
for He is never too busy, and He's never
too late but always on time.
He's always there to hold your hand in the
good times and the bad, all right!
His love for you is more than you can imagine, for it's sublime.

Lean on Him when you feel so all alone and no one seems to care.
Cast all your cares on Him, for He really and truly cares for you.
Never, ever forget to thank Him for His love,
mercy, and grace for you to share.
Always bless, honor, adore, praise, and glorify
His Name and thank Him too.

Jesus is alive forevermore and making intercession for us always.
For now, He is sitting at the right hand
of the power of God to save,
and He's interceding, loving, guiding us by His Holy ways.
Oh, let's come boldly to the throne of grace,
for there is victory over the grave.

Don't Be Weary, My Sister and My Brother

Why do you get weary, my sister and my brother?
Why do you tarry so long?
Instead, why don't you pray and sing?
Don't weep, my brother, for it won't be long.

God is good; God is great.
Let us thank Him all day long.
Let us thank Him for His love,
from way up above.

Kneel to Him in prayer,
for He knows and He cares.
Trust Him today,
and He'll make a way.

Don't be weary, my sister, and my brother.
Don't forget to pray.
Don't forget to sing your song
all the day long.

Day 33

Faith Is the Victory

> Whosoever shall say to this mountain be thou removed, and be cast into the sea and shall not doubt in his heart, but shall believe that those things which he saith shall come to pass; he shall have whatever he saith. Whatsoever things you desire when you pray, believe that you receive them and ye shall have them.
>
> —Mark 11:23–24 (KJV)

To live in victory, demonstrate faith in God in whatever you say and do. "For we walk by faith, not by sight" (2 Corinthians 5:7 KJV). God wants you to live a victorious life by faith. "Now faith is the substance of things hoped for, the evidence of things not seen" (Hebrews 11:1 KJV).

Health care workers provide care and emotional support to their clients; faith is an integral part of their treatment. If you surround your clients with positive, uplifting words and a cheerful environment, they may heal faster and have a better outcome.

One example of Jesus demonstrating faith was when He took the five loaves and two fish from the disciples, broke them, and looked up to heaven and blessed them. Over five thousand men plus women and children ate to the full (and there were leftovers).

John 11:42–44 (KJV) says that Jesus raised Lazarus from the grave after he had been there four days; this is another example of faith in action. "'And I knew that thou hearest me always: but because of the people which stand by I said it, that they may believe that thou hast sent me.' And when he thus had spoken, he cried with a loud voice, 'Lazarus, come forth.' And he that was dead came forth, bound hand and foot with graveclothes: and his face was bound about with a napkin. Jesus saith unto them, 'loose him, and let him go.'" Lazarus was loosed and walked in freedom, alive and well and back in communion with his family and friends. Jesus is the Resurrection and the life. That was faith in action.

If we have faith the size of a mustard seed, we can move mountains. Use your measure of faith, and encourage others to do the same. Faith is the substance of things hoped for, the evidence of things not seen.

A Prayer for Today: Dear Heavenly Father, please increase our faith so that we can live productive and victorious lives as we help those in need. Thank You for hearing and answering our prayers, in the name of Jesus. Amen.

Health Nugget: Avocados are said to be good for dry skin; incorporate them into your diet. They're rich in monounsaturated fats and vitamin E, which promote healthy skin. You can put them in your salads, smoothies, sandwiches, even as a protein side dish.

Hope and Prosperity Gem: Yes, faith is the victory that conquers the world. Go, change your world as you ask God to increase your faith.

Take Time to Seek God

Take time to quietly seek God.
Take time from your hectic schedule.
Take time to seek God,
for He'll help you keep the golden rule.

Ask Him, "What are you saying to my heart?"
Quietly and reverently listen,
for He'll speak through His Word
or whisper words that enlighten.

O Lord, purify our thoughts,
and give us a meek and quiet spirit.
Deepen our hunger for the meaning of the cross,
and strengthen our faith to believe and embrace it.

Growth in Christ: A Must

Our growth in Christ is a must,
for that's His mandate to us.
Add to your faith virtue,
and to virtue add knowledge anew.

To knowledge add self-control,
to self-control add perseverance to your soul.
To perseverance add godliness,
so that we can have genuine success.

Our growth in Christ must continue,
so add to godliness brotherly kindness.
And to brotherly kindness add love,
for love covers a multitude of evils; that is, God's love.

If we do these things and heed the call,
we'll never stumble or fall,
and we'll never be barren or unfruitful
in the knowledge of our Lord Jesus Christ, Who's merciful.

Day 34

Choose the Narrow Way That Leads to Life

> Enter into the narrow gate. For wide is the gate and broad is the road that leads to destruction, and many enter through it. But small is the gate and narrow is the road that leads to life, and only a few find it.
>
> —Matthew 7:13–14 (NIV)

Many people say, "I'm too young; I have more time to enjoy life. I'll go out there and have some fun; when I get older, I'll give my life to the Lord." They say that the road to Christian life is too small, narrow, and restrictive. Instead, they travel the easy, wide, and broad way, which will ultimately lead to destruction. On this wide road, anything goes; no restrictions, do as you please. The consequences of that choice lead to annihilation and regret. So choose Christ, and walk the narrow road, which leads to life, peace, and joy. On this road, Jesus will go with you every step of the way.

He promises that He will hold your right hand with His mighty and righteous right hand of power. You can do it. Just ask the Lord to help keep your focus on Him, trust Him, and obey Him. Endeavor with His help to go where He leads and do what He bids you. If you do these things plus "do justly, and to love mercy, and to walk humbly with thy God," as Micah 6:8 (KJV) purports, you will enjoy the fruit of the spirit and the abundant blessings of the Lord.

Therefore, make that all-important decision to live for Christ. Many youths say they have lots of time because they're young and energetic and have many more years to live and enjoy life. Who told them that they'd live to get old?

Caution: don't wait until tomorrow, for it may be too late. "Now is the accepted time; behold, now is the day of salvation" (2 Corinthians 2:6 KJV). Moses chose to be God's prophet rather than enjoy the fleeting pleasures of sin for a season.

As you make that life-changing decision for Christ, you will find a peace that passes all understanding, a joy beyond compare. You don't have to travel this Christian journey alone. Jesus will always be with you to strengthen and keep you. Why not give your heart to Jesus now? Ask Him to come into your heart and save you and be the Lord of your life. He is waiting and watching and gently knocking at your heart's door, so let Him in.

There are lots of misconceptions about giving your heart and life to Jesus. Some say that this kind of life is too restrictive, too narrow, too binding, and too shallow. That's far from the truth. The Christian life is a sweet life, with Jesus as the Captain and Shepherd. There will be ups and downs, mountains and valleys, good times and bad times, but this is life, in general.

However, with Jesus in the vessel, you could smile at the storm. You have no cause to worry, for Jesus is holding your right hand with His victorious right hand. He'll lead and guide you as you put your trust and confidence in Him. Be assured: The Lord will help you every step of the way.

A Prayer for Today: Dear loving Lord, please help us to recognize the fleeting pleasures of sin and run to You as fast as we can. Remove anything that's blocking the free flow of the Holy Spirit in our lives. Thank You for helping us to be overcomers, in the name of Jesus, we pray. Amen.

Health Nugget: Echinacea is said to reduce cold symptoms. Take as directed at the first sign of symptoms.

Hope and Prosperity Gem: Choose to walk in the light of God's love, and enjoy His abundant blessings.

Choose the Narrow Way

What road will you be finding?
The broad and wide, or the narrow and winding?
The broad and wide road leads to eradication and annihilation.
Choose the narrow and winding road, which
leads to eternal bliss and sin eradication.

Again, the straight broad way leads to death and destruction,
while the narrow and winding way leads to life and liberation.

I choose to walk the narrow road,
with all its trials and heavy load.
I choose to persevere under strife.
I choose Jesus Christ in my life.

Faithful Until He Comes

Let's be faithful and prayerful until He comes.
When He bursts the eastern skies, let's be ready.

While we are waiting and watching,
let's work and be productive.
While we are waiting and watching,
let's worship the Lord and be constructive.

It's never too late to watch and pray,
so let your light shine brightly.
For today may be the day,
so don't take salvation lightly.

Be faithful until death,
and you will a crown of life receive.
Be faithful until the very last breath.
Only trust and believe.

Let's be faithful until Jesus comes,
and let's help each other overcome.

Day 35

God Fights for You

> This is what the Lord says to you: Do not be afraid or discouraged because of this vast army. For the battle is not yours, but God's.
>
> —2 Chronicles 20:15 (NIV)

"And we know that all things work together for good to them that love God, to them who are the called according to his purpose" (Romans 8:28 KJV). God is faithful to His Word. If you're experiencing difficulty caring for your loved one or client, remember: God is with you and will give you the strength you need. When everything seems to be falling apart, and nothing seems to be going right, cry out to Jesus. He is just a prayer away.

When the Israelites were in dire straits, God fought for them. God will also fight for you. He has never lost a battle. An example of God fighting for His children was the battle of Jericho as declared in Joshua 5 and 6 (KJV). The walls came tumbling down after the Israelites encircled them, as instructed, with their trumpets and singers. Immediately, they went forward and took the city as God commanded. That was victory without lifting a finger to fight. God fought for them.

The same God Who fought for the Israelites will fight for you here and now. Just have faith in Him and obey Him without reservation. Say, "Lord, I believe; help my unbelief." Faithful to His inerrant Word, He will help you and give you the victory as He sees fit, according to His will.

God will fight your battles; therefore, you do not have to be anxious or discouraged when bad things happen in your life. Rely on the mercy, power, and goodness of God in stressful situations.

A Prayer for Today: Dear Heavenly Father, I come to You in the precious name of Jesus; thank You for fighting my battles for me. I rest in the protection and shelter of Your wings. Amen.

Health Nugget: Be temperate or moderate in all things. Moderation is the key to health and happiness. Whatever you eat or drink, do everything to honor God.

Hope and Prosperity Gem: Hope in God, and enjoy His most fruitful blessings.

The Secret Place with God

The secret place with God
is where I want to be.
The secret place with God
is where I want Him to see me.

Hide away from the noise.
Hide away and rejoice.
Hide away and pray.
Hide away on your knees today.

Tell Him all your secrets.
Tell Him all your cares.
Tell Him about all your frets
and tell Him all your fears.

Give them to Jesus,
for He cares.
Give them all to Jesus,
for your burdens He shares.

Hide away in your secret place with God.
Read and meditate on His Word reverently.
Hide away in your secret place with God,
and He'll reward you openly.

You Are Special to God

Before you were conceived,
God knew you.
Before you were deceived,
God knew it too.

Before you were born,
He had already walked the sands of time.
Before you were born,
He had your footprints sublime.

Before you even knew yourself,
God had already begun
to shape and mold you like clay,
to prepare you for today.

Before you came to be,
your walls were always before Him, you see.
He molded you in the palms of His hands
so that you'll be ready to preach the Gospel in foreign lands.

You are special to God,
so make Him your Lord.
He will fight your battles;
therefore, stand still because He owns all the cattle.

Day 36

Keep Your Lamp Burning

> Be dressed for service and keep your lamps burning, as though you were waiting for your master to return from the wedding feast.
>
> —Luke 12:35–36 (NIV)

Keep the fire of the Holy Spirit burning wherever you go. Your loved ones and clients are closely observing you. Therefore, you must let your light shine brightly. Light dispels the darkness. John 8:12 (KJV) affirms, "Then spake Jesus unto them, saying, I am the Light of the world: he that followeth Me shall not walk in darkness, but shall have the light of life." Jesus is the source of light within us that would help to lighten the heavy load of the poor and oppressed.

Always stay alert and keep your eyes open when you are providing care. Several years ago, a caregiver fell asleep while on duty. The family took a picture of the worker and presented it to the agency he worked for. The caregiver claimed that he was meditating with his eyes closed. He was reprimanded and removed from the case.

That's why it is so important to keep your eyes open and be attentive when taking care of clients. Let your light shine, and don't hide it under a bushel or sleep on the job. In the same way, be ready, for the coming of the Lord is even at the door.

Keep your lamps burning brightly so that the world can see Jesus in you. Acts of kindness, justice, and mercy help to scatter the darkness. Jesus declares, "You are the salt of the earth; but if the salt loses its flavor, how shall it be seasoned? It is then good for nothing but to be thrown out and trampled underfoot by men. You are the light of the world. A city that is set on a hill cannot be hidden. Nor do they light a lamp and put it under a basket, but on a lampstand, and it gives light to all *who are* in the house. Let your light so shine before men, that they may see your good works and glorify your Father in heaven" (Matthew 5:13-16 NKJV).

Let your life be a testimony of the goodness and love of God the Father through His Son, Christ Jesus. Psalm 119:105 (KJV) says that the "Word is a lamp unto your feet and a light unto your path." Follow that light everywhere you go, and it will lead you the right way.

Perform your duties with the utmost integrity and compassion, and you will be valuable employees and successful citizens. Likewise, you'll enjoy the blessing of the Lord.

A Prayer for Today: Dear Heavenly Father, we need You now more than ever before. You mend the broken-hearted and set the captives free. Please help us to keep our lamps burning brightly for all to see and come to know Thee in the name of Jesus. Amen.

Health Nugget: Are you trying to reduce belly fat? Decrease your carbohydrates, and avoid artificial sweeteners, sugary drinks, and fattening snacks. Refined carbohydrates can spike blood sugar, cause belly fat, and contribute to metabolic syndrome. Instead, choose fruits, vegetables, whole grains, nuts, and beans.

Hope and Prosperity Gem: As you do your best to let your light shine, whether it be on the job or in your daily life, remember that Jesus is coming soon. Live life to the fullest, and do the very best you can each day. There is hope and prosperity for your future, as you place your trust and confidence in the Lord.

Your Word Is a Lamp unto My Feet

God's Word is a lamp unto my feet
and a light unto my path.
Your Word is powerful and sweet
and untouchable from the enemy's wrath.

God's Word is alive.
From it, I would not depart.
My soul and spirit it can divide
for It knows the desires of my heart.

Sometimes, I Feel Downhearted

Sometimes, I feel downhearted.
Sometimes, I feel so blue.
But when I have a little talk with Jesus;
He knows just what to do.

You too may experience pain,
and heartache, and trouble.
So just run to Him today,
and your sadness will crumble.

Keep your lamps burning,
for the Savior's soon returning.
We do not know the day or the hour,
so be ready and serve with boldness and power.

Day 37

Sin Blinds

> The god of this age has blinded the minds of unbelievers so that they cannot see the light of the gospel that displays the glory of Christ, who is the image of God.
>
> —2 Corinthians 4:4 (KJV)

Sin blinds. Sin deceives. Sin hurts. Sin destroys. Sin separates you from God. Sin brings pain and suffering. Sin is enmity against God, our Creator, and Friend.

Because of Adam's sin, sin has plagued the whole world and caused havoc, disease, and death. After Adam and Eve took and ate the forbidden fruit, they immediately realized that they were naked. Disappointed with what they had done, they ran and hid in the garden. The light of God's presence was no longer there to cover their nakedness. Sin had entered their lives.

When God confronted them regarding their sin, Adam and Eve blamed each other, and Eve also blamed the serpent for deceiving her. Because of their decisions, God expelled them from the beautiful Garden of Eden, their home.

Satan had deceived and blinded their eyes to the truth. He is also trying to do the same to us today, but rebuke him in the name of Jesus, and he will flee. He is a cunning and deceitful foe, so keep your eyes on the Lord, for He is good. Romans 2:4 (KJV) states, "Or despiseth thou the riches of his goodness and forbearance and longsuffering; not knowing that the goodness of God leadeth thee to repentance?"

"For the wages of sin is death; but the gift of God is eternal life through Jesus Christ our Lord" (John 6:23 KJV). Sin blinds, but God's love heals and restores. Choose Christ today and always.

A Prayer for Today: Dear Heavenly Father, thank You for loving us the way You do. Open our eyes to see You and only You. Help us to not be blinded by sin and its consequences but to live a holy life, always striving to do the right thing. Thank You, Lord, for helping us today, in Your Holy Name, we pray. Amen.

Health Nugget: Connect with family and friends. Social interaction has been linked to a lower risk of heart disease and increase longevity.

Hope and Prosperity Gem: Purpose in your heart to obey God and do good. Sin will not rule in your heart if you give your life and dreams to the Lord. For everyone born of God overcomes the world.

Don't Wait Another Minute

Don't wait another minute.
Just kneel down and pray,
for if God is in it,
He'll hear what you say.

Don't wait another minute.
Sin can mimic.

Don't waste time.
In the name of Jesus, kneel down and claim it.

Don't waste another minute,
for it just might be too late.
"Too late, too late," may be the cry,
for Jesus may have already passed you by.

Don't wait. Don't procrastinate.
Accept Jesus while it is called today,
for tomorrow may very well be too late.
He is willing and ready to save you right away.

The Fall of Man

That delicious, voluptuous apple, a treat
so beautiful and daunting to behold.
The smell, the aroma so sweet,
the lovely symmetry, taunted Eve's poor soul.

Day after day,
week after week,
month after month,
year after year.

Oh, that forbidden fruit
is looking better and better.
Why can't I touch its root?
If I do, I'll become a trendsetter.

Do not touch or eat this fruit,
for if you, you'll surely die.
That was the Word of the Lord,
and It cannot ever lie.

Here comes the tempter:
"Eve, eat, and you'll realize
that you'll be like God, to know good and evil,
and your eyes will be open without demise."

To the serpent, she kept listening.
Suddenly, she realized the tree was good for food.
The serpent continued his hissing,
"The fruit will make you wise and elevate your mood."

So she picked the fruit and ate thereof,
for she thought it would make her wise.
Her husband Adam took a bite, but it was too late.
"Oh, no, what have we done? We're naked. The serpent lied."

They ran as fast as they could,
sewed fig leaves together,
and made themselves aprons under a hood,
then hid among the trees like a feather.

Fear gripped their hearts for pardon,
for the voice of the Lord God, they heard.
They heard God walking in the garden.
"Adam, where art thou?" asked the Lord God.

"I heard Your voice and was afraid because I was naked."
"Who told you that you were naked? Did
you eat the forbidden fruit?"
"I did, Lord," said Adam.

Adam accused Eve, his gem.
Eve accused the serpent, her enemy,
for the serpent beguiled them,
and they lost their liberty and changed their destiny.

Sin blinds and causes separation from God for all to see.
But Jesus broke the power of sin and set us free.
Genesis 2 (KJV)

Day 38

Touch Not, Taste Not, Handle Not

> Touch not; taste not; handle not; which all are to perish with the using; after the commandments and doctrines of men? Which things have indeed a shew of wisdom in will worship, and humility, and neglecting of the body: not in any honour to the satisfying of the flesh.
>
> —Colossians 2:21–23 (KJV)

God, in His love and mercy and grace, always warns His children. The warnings are real and done in love. God wants you to enjoy life to the fullest and be abundant and prosperous. The enemy of your soul, on the other hand, wants to destroy you. He comes in as an angel of light, with subtlety and deception. The devil doesn't approach you as an enemy but as an angel of light.

Miss Yanni, a Christian health care professional, had been warned over and over as she read the Bible not to touch, taste, or handle anything that God condemns. Despite the frequent warnings, she yielded to temptation, which caused her life to spiral downhill. From that traumatic experience, Miss Yanni clearly understood that

God's Word is accurate and the warnings were for her good. The Lord wanted her to enjoy life to the fullest.

God tempts no one. The temptation stems from one's desires. "When lust is conceived, it brings forth sin: and sin, when it is finished, bringeth forth death" (James 1:15 KJV). Disobedience to the dictates of the Bible can thwart one's dreams and aspirations, family unity, peace, and joy. The lesson here is to obey the Lord and follow Him.

The apostle John continues with his warning: "My little children, these things write I unto you, that ye sin not. And if any man sin, we have an advocate with the Father, Jesus Christ the righteous: and he is the propitiation for our sins: and not for ours only, but also for the sins of the whole world" (1 John 2:1–2 KJV).

God's love is real. Obey His commands and live.

A Prayer for Today: Dear Lord, Your Word is inerrant, and Your warnings are always for our good. Help us, Lord, to be obedient and touch not, handle not, and taste not the things You have forbidden. Thank You for helping us to walk in freedom and victory, in the name of Jesus, we pray. Amen.

Health Nugget: Cranberry juice could help in the treatment of a urinary tract infection and reduce its severity; take as directed.

Hope and Prosperity Gem: Failing but coming back even stronger is what God wants for His children. Don't give up. When you fall, get back up, brush yourself off, and repent. God will forgive you. There is hope for your future.

One Life to Live

We only have one life,
so let's make the best of it.
Living a life without strife
can only be done with the help of the Holy Spirit.

Give your life to Jesus now.
Let Him have control.
Give your life to Jesus now,
for He'll give you eternal life that will never grow old.

Whether you are old or young,
Jesus wants you as His servant.
He'll give you a new song;
praise Him, honor Him, and worship Him, and be fervent.

Trust and Obey

Trust and obey, for Jesus is the Rock of the Ages,
the foundation on which we stand.
Even though our enemy rages,
our foundation will always stand.

Rest your head on His breast.
Lean on His everlasting arm,
and He'll give you what's best.
There's no reason for alarm.

Day 39

Dream Big

> Ye are of God, little children, and have overcome them: because greater is he that is in you, than he that is in the world.
>
> —1 John 4:4 (KJV)

God's dreams for you are more significant than your own dreams. They are for your protection, peace, and joy. Dream big, and do all things to the honor and glory of the Lord. When you do this, you'll be honoring God with the works of your hands, and He will prosper you.

Many health care workers and caregivers have challenging assignments, especially when covering staff shortages. I've been there, and it was very taxing to my body. I needed to get lots of rest to recuperate from the stress and long, exhausting hours.

Jesus is our Good Shepherd and cares for His sheep. If one sheep is lost and escaped from the sheepfold, Jesus Himself will go in search of it. When He finds the sheep, He'll lovingly embrace him in His arms and take him back to the sheepfold. Jesus also pursues you. When the sheep stray, He will gently lead them back into the sheepfold. The sheep will not run away from the Shepherd, for he recognizes His voice; a stranger he would not follow.

As a health care worker or caregiver, dream big, and do your best in all your endeavors. Get the education and skills needed to perform your job with precision and integrity. And no good thing will the Lord deny you if you walk honestly, act humbly, love mercy, and do justly.

Stay focused, set realistic goals, and work diligently toward achieving them. With God's help, you could overcome challenges and stand firm on the principles of integrity. Dreaming big can also enhance the quality of your life, as you help others in the process.

A Prayer for Today: Dear Heavenly Father, help us to dream big, for we are Your people and the sheep of Your pasture. You always want the very best for Your children, so help us to seek You first and be all You've called us to be, in the name of Jesus. Amen.

Health Nugget: Benefits of a positive attitude include the following: improved health, reduced stress and anxiety, fewer sick call-outs, and more stamina.

Hope and Prosperity Gem: There is hope, love, and abundant blessings in your future, God willing. Believe by faith and give God all the praise, honor, and glory, for He is worthy to be praised.

Hold on to Your Dreams

Hold on to your dreams.
Never give up.
Capture your heart's desire,
and never give up.

Don't let them steal your joy.
Don't let them quench your dreams.
Fight if you may,
but hold on to them tenaciously every day.

You are worth loving and hugging.
Don't give up. Hold on to your dreams.

Don't let them tie you down.
Don't let their mouths bind you.
Don't let their lips mar what you've sown.
Don't let their lies hinder you.

For you are special in God's eyes.
You are the apple of His eyes for sure.
You are the golden apple encased by God, so wise,
and you're precious in His sight; that's pure.

Day 40

A Merry Heart Is Good Medicine

> A merry heart does good, like medicine, but a broken spirit dries the bones.
>
> —Proverbs 17:22 (NKJV)

Laugh yourself to good health. Laughter is said to be the internal jogging of your vital organs. The great thing about laughter is that it's good medicine, and it's free for all to enjoy. Reap the benefits, which are wellness and vitality.

Envy, on the other hand, is rottenness to the bone. When you laugh, especially a deep belly laugh, it releases endorphins, relieving pain more effectively than morphine.

God loves you so much that He has blessed you with excellent medicine that could keep you active and healthy. Studies have confirmed the many benefits of laughter: it helps to relieve stress and anxiety, decreases chronic diseases, gives a sense of wellness, decreases high blood pressure by causing vasodilation of the vessels, promotes heart health, increases circulation, decreases arthritic aches and pain, and decreases the severity of migraines.

As you care for your clients and loved ones, remember to laugh. Yes, sometimes even laugh at yourself. It's an effective medicine for you to partake as often as you desire. God has given it to you, so enjoy and use it often.

Laugh at least fifteen to twenty times a day. That should keep you energetic, vibrant, enthusiastic, and healthy.

As you continue to keep your eyes fixed on Jesus, you'll have the victory over temptation and sin. If you feel sad and discouraged because of the pressures of life, run to Jesus. Call out to Him, "Jesus, Jesus, Jesus, I need You now more than ever before. Please help me. I'm having a difficult time coping with the pressures and demands of life."

As you cry out to Him, He'll help you: "For the Lord God is a sun and shield: The Lord will give grace and glory: no good thing will He withhold from them that walk uprightly" (Psalm 84:11 KJV).

Thank You, Lord, for hearing and answering my prayers. I love You, Lord. Thank You for loving me with a steadfast love.

Finally, health care workers and caregivers: love and embrace your clients and loved ones, with outstretched arms, just like the Lord.

A Prayer for Today: Dear Lord, You said that a merry heart does good like medicine. Help us to trust and obey You; we believe by faith that You have blessed us with cheerful and joyful hearts. Show us how to maintain health and wellness and live useful, productive lives. Thank You, heavenly Father, for hearing and answering our prayers in the name of Jesus, we pray. Amen.

Health Nugget: Laugh your way to good health. Cast all your cares, tension, and anxieties at the foot of the cross, and leave them there, for Jesus cares for you. Moreover, He will brighten your day and give you peace of mind. Rejoice in the Lord always, and be thankful for what He has given you. Again, I say, rejoice.

Hope and Prosperity Gem: When the Lord fills our hearts with joy and peace, He can lead us through the most challenging situations and give us a sense of hope and purpose. Such confidence comes from personally knowing Jesus as Savior and Lord. Enjoy the abundant blessings of the Lord. You were born to be a winner with a merry heart.

A Merry Heart Is Like Medicine

God gives us the opportunity to impart His love,
if only we are keen to listen.
His still small voice, like a dove,
will make our merry hearts glisten.

God arranges the affairs of man
to fulfill His plans.
Be ready as a soldier, faithful and true,
because God is counting on you.

Feed the flock of God,
whether in small or big ways.
Feed the flock of God with your life of praise,
and remember He works in mysterious ways.

So laugh as hard as you wish and as often as you can,
for that is like medicine to your body and
soul, for Jesus is the Son of Man.

Laugh Your Way to Victory in Jesus

Hallelujah, the children of God have the victory
in Jesus, the Resurrected King of kings.
He's also Lord of lords, the Great I AM,
the Mighty Conqueror, the Lion of Judah, the Mighty King,
and God's Spotless Holy and Righteous Lamb.
So we can laugh our way to health, for
Jesus is our soon-coming King.

Oh, come to Jesus while you have life.
Oh, come to Jesus while you have hope.
Oh, come to Jesus, for He will save you from strife.
Oh, come to Jesus now, and He'll give you a
merry heart full of peace and hope.

Notes

Notes

Notes

Notes

Lightning Source UK Ltd.
Milton Keynes UK
UKHW011159091219
355041UK00002B/432/P